One Foot in Eden

The International Library of Group Psychotherapy and Group Process

Therapeutic Communities Section

Section Editors

R. D. Hinshelwood
Consultant Psychotherapist
St Bernard's Hospital, Southall, Middlesex

Nick Manning
Lecturer in Social Policy and Administration
University of Kent

One Foot in Eden

A Sociological Study of the Range of Therapeutic Community Practice

Michael Bloor
MRC Medical Sociology Unit
University of Glasgow

Neil McKeganey
Social Paediatric and Obstetric Research Unit
University of Glasgow

Dick Fonkert
Austerlitz
Netherlands

Routledge
London and New York

First published in 1988 by
Routledge
11 New Fetter Lane, London EC4P 4EE

Published in the USA by
Routledge, Chapman and Hall, Inc.
in association with Methuen Inc.
29 West 35th Street, New York, NY 10001

Set in Times, 10/12 point
by Witwell Ltd, Southport
and printed in Great Britain
by T. J. Press (Padstow) Ltd,
Padstow, Cornwall

Library of Congress Cataloging in Publication Data
Bloor, Michael.
One foot in Eden : a sociological study of the range of therapeutic community practice / Michael Bloor, Neil McKeganey, Dick Fonkert.
p. cm. – (The International library of group psychotherapy and group process. Therapeutic communities series)
Bibliography: p.
Includes index.
1. Social psychiatry. 2. Mental health facilities.
3. Psychiatric hospitals. I. McKeganey, Neil P. II. Fonkert, Dick. III. Title. IV. Series
RC455.B554 1988
362.2'1 – dc 19 88–330

British Library Cataloguing in Publication Data
Bloor, Michael
One foot in Eden : a sociological study of the range of therapeutic community practice.
1. Therapeutic communities
I. Title II. McKeganey, Neil P. 1955–
III. Fonkert, Dick
362.2'0425

ISBN 0-415-00822-0

To Gordon Horobin 1926–1987

Contents

Acknowledgments

This comparative study was long in the making: the first of the component studies was begun more than ten years ago. Along the way we have incurred many debts which we are happy to acknowledge here. Our work would have been stillborn without the kind cooperation of the members (staff and residents) of the eight therapeutic communities in which our component studies were conducted. We only have permission to mention one of these communities by name – Aberdeen's Ross Clinic day hospital. Financial support was provided by the Medical Research Council (Michael Bloor) and the Economic and Social Research Council (Neil McKeganey). We wish to thank the past and present directors of the Medical Research Council's Medical Sociology Unit (Raymond Illsley and Sally MacIntyre) and the director of Glasgow University's Social Paediatric and Obstetric Research Unit (Andrew Boddy) for their institutional support, their advice and their encouragement. We also wish to thank Ilja Maso of the University of Leiden for his advice and encouragement on one of the component studies.

We are grateful to the editor of *Sociology of Health and Illness* and to Basil Blackwell Ltd for permission to reprint from McKeganey, N. and Bloor, M. (1987), 'Teamwork, information control and therapeutic effectiveness', *Sociology of Health and Illness*, vol. 9, pp. 154–78. We are grateful to the editor of the *Journal of Adolescence*, Academic Press, and the Association for the Psychiatric Study of Adolescents for permission to reprint material from Bloor, M. (1986), 'Problems of therapeutic community practice in two halfway houses for disturbed adolescents: a comparative sociological study', *Journal of Adolescence*, vol. 9, pp. 29–48. We are grateful to the editor of the *International Journal of Sociology and*

Social Policy and to Barmarick Publications Ltd for permission to reprint material from Bloor, M. and McKeganey, N. (1986), 'Conceptions of therapeutic work in therapeutic communities', *International Journal of Sociology and Social Policy*, vol. 6, pp. 68–79. We are also grateful to W. H. Auden's executors, to Faber and Faber Ltd and to Random House Inc. for permission to quote from 'Get there if you can . . .' in *The English Auden: poems, essays, and dramatic writings 1927–1939*, London, Faber and Faber, and in Collected Poems, edited by Edward Mendelson, New York, Random House.

Many colleagues have given us comments on our analyses of the component studies – David Armstrong, David Brien, Sarah Cunningham-Burley, Jon Gabe, Douglas Haldane, Robert Harris, Bob Harrison, Jim McIntosh, Ken Morrice, Lindsay Prior, Barbara Rawlings, Victor Sharp, Phil Strong and Gareth Williams. The series editors – Bob Hinshelwood and Nick Manning – have commented on our comparative analysis. Andy Rigby has commented on Chapter Three, and Sarah Cunningham-Burley on the appendix. Anne Gould, Kim Macindoe, Edna MacIntyre, Jean Money, Gill Sinclair and Janet Watson typed various drafts of our manuscript. Irene Hind quickly and efficiently compiled the index.

Our greatest debt is to Gordon Horobin, to whom this book is dedicated. Shortly after it was agreed to dedicate it to him, Gordon suddenly died. We consider ourselves lucky to have worked with Gordon for as long as we did. There are not many in the academic world who combine the qualities of friend and colleague as effectively as Gordon was able to. For that and much more he will be greatly missed.

Introduction

We begin with a bit of tub-thumping. We cannot be anything other than surprised at our achievement in putting together ethnographies of therapeutic work in eight different therapeutic communities: we know of no other published sociological project (on therapeutic communities or any other institution or social phenomenon) that has incorporated so many different ethnographic studies. Indeed, it is the conventional wisdom in sociology that the 'qualitative' research methods we employed must sacrifice breadth of coverage for depth of coverage: in-depth ethnographies of institutions are considerably more time-consuming than survey and interview methods, and such ethnographies cannot be repeated in a series of institutions within the three-year time-limit that funding agencies normally expect of sociological research. The judgment of Tizard and his colleagues is both representative and authoritative: 'it is normally impracticable for a research worker to provide detailed qualitative descriptions of more than one or two institutions' (Tizard et al., 1975, p. 2).

We have managed to avoid this constraint because the eight communities described in this book were the foci of six different individual studies (two of them comparative). Because all these individual studies involved the collection of similar (largely participant observational) data on aspects of the same broad topic (the treatment process), it has been possible to reuse these data for a single comparative study. This was not happenstance, but a strategy that was developed at an early stage in the study: the locations for the later individual studies were deliberately selected to encompass a range of therapeutic community practice.

There are many different kinds of institutions with claims to the title of therapeutic community; they differ radically in their staffing, their clientele, their social organisation and their approaches to treatment. There is no such thing as a single 'representative' therapeutic community. If one wishes to portray the nature of therapeutic community work, this can only be undertaken within a comparative framework since a central feature of therapeutic community work is its variability between different communities.

The eight communities included in our study were as follows. The first two, 'Faswells' and 'Ravenscroft', were two small residential treatment units (studied by McKeganey) located within traditional psychiatric hospitals. They were staffed by psychiatrists, psychiatric nurses and various ancillary professionals and treated mainly neurotic or personality-disordered patients in group therapy programmes set within democratic and permissive treatment regimes; they followed a model of therapeutic community practice pioneered by the doyen of therapeutic communities in Britain, Maxwell Jones (Jones, 1952, 1968, 1982). Such hospital communities are subject to considerable fluctuations over time in daily practice and effectiveness – indeed, it has been argued that cyclical crises are native to the therapeutic community method (Rapoport, 1960). Accordingly, we have chosen two hospital communities experiencing contrasting fortunes.

Our third community, and the only non-residential one, was Aberdeen's Ross Clinic day hospital (studied by Bloor). This community also followed a treatment approach of Maxwell Jones-type group therapy, but the majority of patients were day patients, returning to their homes in the evenings and at weekends.

Although in Britain it is the Maxwell Jones-type model which, more than any other, is popularly associated with the term 'therapeutic community', in America the term normally connotes quite a different model of practice, that of the 'concept house' for the treatment of drug addicts. Basing their approach on the Synanon 'concept' (Synanon being the first of these communities; see Yablonsky, 1965), the concept houses are closed and controlled environments where staff (usually themselves ex-addicts) programme residents through a taxing schedule of activities organised within an elaborate hierarchy of statuses. Our fourth community was a Dutch concept house, studied by Fonkert.

Our fifth community was a Camphill Rudolf Steiner School, studied by McKeganey. It was part of the Camphill movement, a world-wide network of communities caring for mentally handicapped and disturbed children (and more recently for mentally handicapped adults and for the elderly), inspired by the Christianised theosophical teachings of Rudolf Steiner (1861–1925). All the staff (called co-workers) lived and worked communally (no salaries) with the children in large houses set within a model village on its own secluded estate.

'Parkneuk' (studied by Bloor) was our sixth community, also communally organised and a secular off-shoot of the Camphill movement. But whereas the population of McKeganey's Camphill community was around 370, that of Parkneuk never numbered more than fourteen. Parkneuk was a community that came close to the foster-family model of care for the mentally handicapped and disturbed, a model that has long been followed in several European countries (Wing, 1957; Strole, 1977).

Our last two communities were 'Ashley' and 'Beeches' (studied by Bloor), halfway houses run by the same charitable trust and catering for similar client groups (disturbed adolescents). Ashley's permissive regime had its ancestry in the Maxwell Jones model, whereas Beeches' attempts to programme residents' behaviour within a hierarchical structure bore resemblances to the concept house model.

It seems likely that questions will be asked about the representativeness of our sample of eight communities. We have chosen a 'theoretical sample' to embrace the range of community practice, but it may be argued that we should have cast our net wider. Perhaps we should have included an example of a penal institution run along therapeutic community lines, such as Grendon prison (Barratt, 1978), or the Barlinnie Special Unit (Boyle, 1977), or various List D schools (Walter, 1978). Equally, it may be argued that we ought to have studied St Mungo's or one of the Cyrenian communities set up to assist those on skid row (Rigby, 1974, pp. 143–4; Leach and Wing, 1980). Perhaps, in addition to the Camphill community, we should have included another residential school community like Peper Harrow or the Mulberry Bush School (Dockar-Drysdale, 1968), or another religious community such as one of the Communités de L'Arche (Clarke, 1974). Possibly we should have done work at the Cassel Hospital, where another pioneer, Dr. Thomas Main, has developed with his colleagues a unique synthesis of group therapy and individual psychoanalysis.

It is right that such questions should be asked, and qualifications be added to our claim to have sampled the range of practice. However, we would ask questioners to bear three points in mind. First, the exigencies and constraints of research work have been such as to make it impossible for us to add further observational studies to our present (already considerable) total. Second, although it may be arguable that there are types of practice missing from our sample, we have nevertheless included six seemingly different types of community in the sample and also looked at variations in practice within given types of community. And finally, it should be recognised that there is no determinate answer to the question of how many types of community there are: as with any social phenomenon, the closer the inspection of the phenomenon, the more the variation that is apparent. Had we found the time and resources to embrace additional communities such as Grendon Prison or Cassel Hospital, it might still be asked why we had not included in our sample a local authority day centre as well as a day hospital, or why we did not include halfway house communities catering for client groups other than disturbed adolescents. There is no self-evident cut-off point for the sample and the one we have adopted was, of necessity, essentially arbitrary.

So far we have skirted round the question of how one actually defines a therapeutic community. The issue is a tricky one, not least because of the disparate character of the communities themselves. It is also an issue upon which much ink has already been spilt. As McKeganey (1982) has pointed out elsewhere, each type of community has evolved distinctive organisational features, so that a definition which adequately describes one such organisational type is bound to exclude another type, and vice versa. Thus, Clark (1965) tried to distinguish between a 'therapeutic community approach' and the 'therapeutic community proper', reserving the latter term for the Maxwell Jones-type hospital communities. But those speaking out on behalf of the concept houses have disputed whether the principles of 'democracy' and 'permissiveness', upon which Jones's practice was founded, are necessarily central to therapeutic communities, and have stressed the importance of all community members having similar histories if the staff/patient distinction is to be overcome (most senior concept house members are themselves ex-addicts). Similarly, we have heard Camphill members question whether a true community is possible where some within the community receive salaries for caring for other community members (see Weihs, 1975, *passim*). However, it is generally recognised that some divergence in models of the therapeutic community is necessary and inevitable, since there must be horses for courses and the courses of therapeutic communities are so diverse: 'what is appropriate for the ward of a mental hospital may be out of place in a school for delinquents' (Morrice, 1968, p. 126).

In this climate of tolerance many have adopted (and quoted) Jones's minimal definition: 'there is, as yet, no one model of a therapeutic community and all that is intended is that it should mobilise the interest, skills and enthusiasms of staff and patients and give them sufficient freedom of action to create their own optimal treatment and living conditions' (Jones, 1962, p. 73). Others have abandoned attempts at definition and accorded the name therapeutic community to any institution that claims it – Clark has now adopted this position (Clark, 1977). One commentator has treated the problem as an exemplar of the wider philosophical difficulty of achieving an adequate definition of any phenomenon, insofar as the act of definition involves the selection of supposedly central properties from an infinitely extendable list of possible descriptors, and any selection made will be a value judgment, essentially arbitrary, and open to disagreement and dispute (Rawlings, 1981).

We will add our own (minimal) definition to the existing stockpile, not because we dissent from any of these previous judgments, or because we believe we can produce a universally acceptable definition where others have failed, but because our definition will signal to readers the approach we mean to adopt in comparing our eight communities. We wish to focus not on features of the social *organisation* of communities as such, but rather on the *act* of therapy, on everyday therapeutic work. We conceive of therapeutic work as a cognitive activity which can transform any mundane event in the community by *redefining* that event in the light of some therapeutic paradigm; thus an event may be redefined as showing responsibility, or seeking out a new and less pathogenic way of relating to others, or whatever, with the precise nature of the redefinition (and of the paradigm on which it is based) varying from community to community. To so redefine an everyday event as an occasion or a topic for therapy sets it apart and transforms it, much as the profane is transformed into the sacred by religious belief and ceremony; a simple act like cleaning the toilets or mending a leaking sink is invested with new meaning and held up as relevant to the cleaner's recovery or rehabilitation. Any and every event and activity in the therapeutic community is potentially open to such redefinition; there is no nook or cranny of resident life that is not open to scrutiny and potentially redefinable in therapeutic terms. As a result the ward, house, or unit in question can no longer be conceived of either as a neutral backcloth for professionally administered therapies, or as a deviant subculture subverting the professional regime; the act of redefinition recreates the everyday social life of that ward, house or unit as an agency of therapy in its own right. It is with this act of redefinition that we will be concerned in this book, with plotting its variable incidence, features, and manifestations from community to community. We therefore define therapeutic communities as locales where any and every mundane event and activity is potentially open to redefinition in terms of a therapeutic paradigm, with the nature of the paradigm and of the redefinition varying from community to community.

The act of redefinition does not just imaginatively transform the patient's environment, reconstituting it as an agency of therapy, redefinitions also play a direct therapeutic role in that they cumulatively alter the perceptions of residents, perceptions both of themselves and of their social world. This process of perceptual change is often called 'social learning' by therapeutic community practitioners and 'reality construction' by sociologists (Berger and Luckmann, 1967). The way in which redefinitions are communicated to residents will vary between communities: in some communities, for example, an important method will be reality confrontation – the reflection back to the resident of his/her conduct (Morrice, 1979). To a differing extent in different communities, the repetition of the redefinition by both staff and fellow residents may lead to its eventual acceptance and assimilation by the resident – the redefinition becomes a taken-for-granted, 'objective' fact of the resident's life. As residents learn to account for their past and present behaviour in terms of the assimilated redefinition, then their behaviour is reconstituted by that redefinition, becomes that redefinition – such is the power of language to constitute reflexively the reality it purports to describe. Just as the revised history which it was Winston Smith's occupation to rewrite in Orwell's *1984* became the true and only history, so also patients may become the persons whose actions and feelings they have learnt to redefine. The act of redefinition is thus the motor of therapy. These and other themes are the focus of subsequent chapters.

In Chapter 1 we provide an historical context for our subsequent discussion by briefly outlining the development of therapeutic community approaches to treatment and care. Although there are already available a number of very useful historical accounts, most of these concentrate upon the development of communities within residential psychiatric institutions. By contrast we shall focus upon the use of therapeutic community techniques in a diverse range of settings, in which quite different beliefs about the meaning of health, illness, care, and treatment are often found.

In Chapter 2 of this survey we try to convey a sense of what life and work was like in each of our eight communities. The critic Northrop Frye, discussing Utopian literature like Sir Thomas More's original *Utopia*, Bellamy's *Looking Backward* and Huxley's *Island*, has commented unfavourably on the overly rational accounts of those perfect societies where a tolerant guide solemnly explains to the novice/visitor/author how every mundane or puzzling event that they witness in fact plays its part in The Harmonious Whole. This rational explanation of every minute feature, satirised by Frye as the State Intourist Guide literary device (Frye, 1967), is equally discernible in some therapeutic community practitioner literature which abounds with hyperbolic statements such as '... even mundane tasks such as fridge defrosting and toilet cleaning were viewed as learning situations requiring certain skills to achieve the desired result.' By trying to recapture our own initial, unformed impressions of the communities as incoming researchers we try to avoid the laboured earnestness of Frye's Soviet guides and give a sense of what life was like within each of the settings.

In Chapter 3 we erect a distinction between the communities in the nature of their everyday therapeutic work. On the one hand, we distinguish communities where the main medium for behavioural change is reality confrontation – the repeated reflection back to the resident by both staff and fellow residents of their view of his or her conduct, in the hope that he or she will eventually accept the collective view of that conduct as inappropriate, and seek to change it. On the other hand, we can distinguish those communities where the main medium for behavioural change is a kind of social engineering: the careful manipulation and control of the social environment of the resident together with close supervision and didactic, step-wise instruction of resident activity up to the point where new, non-pathogenic patterns of behaviour are mastered and adopted. In the first type of community the object of therapeutic work is to make the resident the observer of his or her own behaviour; the resident sees and accepts the 'looking glass self' (Cooley, 1983) reflected back by the rest of the community, and concurs with the community in the view that he or she should adopt a different pattern of behaviour. Within those communities the aim of inducing behavioural change is constantly before the resident and part of the work of therapy consists in repeatedly stressing the desirability of such change. This contrasts with the second type of community, where the therapist attempts to achieve his or her aim in an instrumental fashion, by maintaining a controlled environment for the resident and supervising his or her performance in such a way that new behaviours are called forth willy-nilly, simply by dint of performing those tasks in that environment. The therapist's aims are thus achieved obliquely by his or her instruments and remain largely or wholly hidden from the resident.

Useful as this distinction may be, it is one which should not be overdrawn since in practice all communities engage, to varying degrees, in both types of therapeutic work. What is important for our purposes is to chart the different emphasis different communities attach to these different types of therapeutic work. Thus the Camphill community, for example, places considerable emphasis on creating around the handicapped child the kind of social environment which will allow the spirit that lies within the handicapped child to achieve its spiritual purpose: anthroposophists (followers of Rudolf Steiner) believe that each spirit *chooses* to be reborn within a handicapped body in order to obtain some definite and individual spiritual goal, and so the therapist's function is to engineer an appropriate social environment in order for that spiritual development to occur. Although such an approach would indicate a purely instrumental approach to therapeutic community practice, in fact the residential staff (co-workers) who lived alongside the children often sought to involve them in common daily household tasks and could frequently be heard confronting inappropriate behaviour and demanding changes in child behaviour if only to ensure that necessary household tasks were completed. In practice, then, as we will aim to show, every community employs a mix of therapeutic approaches, although we can map substantial inter-community variations in the emphasis accorded each approach.

In Chapter 4 we turn our attention to the way in which different communities conceptualise different notions of resident progress. All communities recognise different statuses among residents – senior and junior residents, neophytes and graduands. The movement of residents through these different statuses may be formal or informal, a ceremonial announcement in a community meeting, or a private and fleeting staff assessment in the course of laying the dinner tables. In either case these status rankings are an embodiment of notions of resident progress. In different communities progress will be visualised and recognised in different ways. In some communities pre-eminent in the notion of progress is the acquisition by residents of an ability to account for their individual and collective behaviour in ways which accord with and sustain the dominant ideology (we use the term non-pejoratively) of the community. In other communities progress is judged more by the standard of increasing resident competence in the performance of given tasks and in social situations, competence which is promoted by didactic instruction and by meticulous planning and control of the resident's environment. These contrasting notions of resident progress may be tied to our earlier distinction between communities which proceed largely by reality confrontation and those which proceed largely by instrumental intervention.

Chapter 5 is concerned with two related topics, that of variations in the audience for redefinitions and that of resident resistance to redefinitions. Once again we find a broad distinction between reality-confronting and instrumental communities, this time in the typical audience for expressed redefinitions: whilst residents are the main audience for redefinitions in reality-confronting communities, fellow staff are the main audience in instrumental communities.

Group (as opposed to individual) treatment methods are only possible if individual residents are held to experience common problems and to benefit from common situations. Yet such a communal orientation can never be total; the framework of treatment must also be able to embrace individual needs. The extent to which residents' problems may be treated as common is variable and potentially subject to dispute. In instrumental communities this intermingling of individual and collective treatment is achieved by prior 'backstage' planning by staff members. In reality-confronting communities it is achieved, in part, by shifts back and forth in the audience for redefinitions between the individual and collectivity, and in part by instructing residents to see parallels between their own situation and that of their fellows. The audience for any given redefinition is not fixed but rather is extensible.

This ambiguity in the matter of the audience for redefinitions alerts us to the fact that redefinitions of events may be avoided or contested by residents. In their differing ways all communities seek to overcome rigid distinctions between staff and residents, and in all communities important therapeutic work is undertaken by fellow residents as well as staff. Nevertheless, as in all institutions, inequalities in power relations are a routine fact of social life in therapeutic communities.

There is a power relationship which is manifested most clearly in the surveillance staff exercise over residents. It is only if events and activities are open to inspection that therapists have the potential to redefine mundane events: surveillance must precede redefinition. Not surprisingly, then, behaviour by residents which seeks to contest that power relationship is not confined to contesting staff redefinitions, but is also concerned with resisting surveillance by concealing occurrences from the staff gaze.

Thus resident reaction to subordinate status often takes the form of resistance to therapy, and relations of power between superordinates and subordinates are irremediably confounded with relations of therapy between therapists and residents. There is an inevitable and tragic tendency for all subordinate revolt to be viewed as pathognomonic by staff, and for all superordinate therapeutic initiatives to be viewed by residents as attempts at domination. Ken Kesey's *One Flew Over The Cuckoo's Nest* (1962) remains the most forceful statement of the patient's viewpoint in this mismatch of perspectives.

The forms of individual and collective resident resistance and the forms of staff counteraction varied between communities. In Chapter 5 we map these different techniques of power and resistance across our eight communities.

The focus of our sixth chapter is the influence of external constraints upon therapeutic community practice. One aspect of this topic that has received a good deal of attention is the relationship between those psychiatric units run along therapeutic community lines and the staff and administration of the larger psychiatric hospitals in which many of those communities are based. In fact, the decline in numbers of such communities has, on occasion, been attributed to their sometimes uneasy relations with their host institutions. By adopting an inter-community framework of analysis we shall show how difficulties in external relationships that have apparently had a deleterious effect on practice in some communities have also been experienced in other communities with far less damaging consequences. It will be evident that the adoption of certain practices may serve to minimise problems of external constraints. And it will also be clear that what are in effect internal difficulties in the operation of certain communities may be ascribed mistakenly to external problems.

In our concluding chapter we draw out what we feel are the implications of our study for sociologists, for therapeutic community practitioners, and for a general readership. For sociologists we identify six formal properties or principles of therapeutic work – that therapeutic work is reflexive, interpretative, interventionist, dominating, selective, and subject to habituation. Each of these properties except the first is differentially extensible, so the different communities in our study can be distinguished in, for example, the degree to which therapeutic work is dominating, or is subject to habituation. We consider the merits of our conceptualisation of therapeutic work relative to other conceptualisations found in the sociological literature and we suggest it might form a suitable basis for analyses of therapeutic work from a comparative perspective in other areas of medical practice. Moreover, many of the social processes we depict within therapeutic communities are to be found within a multitude of social settings, so we hope for a wider relevance for, say, our analysis of the induction of new members and their instruction in new ways of behaving and of interpreting each others' actions.

For practitioners we have chosen to highlight some aspects of practice (seven in all) currently found in just one or two communities in our sample but which might, with some advantage, be adopted more widely. These are practices which might increase the effectiveness of therapeutic work in various different ways – by combating resident institutionalisation, by reducing defaulting rates, and so on. We would not argue their universal applicability, nor can we claim a definite relationship with increased practice effectiveness – this would demand controlled evaluative studies and such studies are probably an impossibility in therapeutic communities. Our position is simply that all comparative studies are, of their nature, relevant to the issue of evaluation; we have felt duty-bound to make explicit certain aspects of practice which are implicitly approbated by comparisons. We have not aimed to produce a recipe book for successful therapeutic community practice, but only to draw attention to contrasting attempted solutions to comparable problems.

Of course, we also hope that the various descriptions of practice themselves will appeal to practitioners. Only a few of the existing studies deal with more than one community and none of them adopt the particular comparative approach followed here. Not only will we be providing reports on a much wider range of practice than has been available hitherto, we will also be able to elucidate common themes and difficulties shared between different communities.

There is also material here to interest a more general readership. By entitling this survey *One Foot in Eden* we wish to highlight the Utopian element which we feel is a central part of all therapeutic community practice. We use the term Utopia not in any derogatory sense, but to point to the way in which all communities seek to draw new residents into a new world of caring relationships and to contrast these with the old world from which the new resident has come, and of which he or she was in some sense a casualty.

This contrast between the new resident's Utopian future and redeemable past has an obvious utility for therapy, and the same Utopian element engenders a high degree of commitment among therapeutic community staff and patients. As we shall see in subsequent chapters, the process of inducting new residents may, in some communities, parallel religious conversion, leaving all but the neophyte resident with a high commitment to the community and the treatment process. It is this potential for the transformation of self which may explain the interest in therapeutic communities shown by the radicals of the sixties and early seventies. It was not just humanitarian revolt against the horrors of the custodial mental hospitals which served as a spur, nor the democratic and egalitarian ethos of some of the new communities, nor yet the charm for disaffected adolescents of Laing's diatribes against the authoritarian family, but the possibility of personal and collective liberation from a supposedly pathogenic society.

In our conclusion we assess the potential of therapeutic communities for reducing what Ivan Illich, libertarian critic of the medical enterprise, has called 'structural iatrogenesis' – the creation of sickness through the expropriation of the power of individuals and collectivities to heal themselves (Illich, 1975, p. 165).

We include an appendix on research methods. The appendix will embrace discussions of the drawing of our sample of communities, of data-collection, and of methods of analysis.

Two final points need to be made. First, therapeutic communities, like all institutions, change over time and some of the data used in this study were collected ten years ago. We are aware that many of our study communities have undergone considerable changes since fieldwork was completed. We should make it clear that our analyses only pertain to the communities as they existed during the periods of our fieldwork.

Finally, a note on nomenclature: some of the communities we have studied are referred to by pseudonyms and others by their true names

– this reflects the preferences of each community's members at the time when the component studies were undertaken. In all quoted fieldnotes and reported anecdotes names and, where necessary, certain background circumstances have been changed to prevent identification. Different communities designate 'staff' and 'patients' by different names which reflect different conceptions of staff-patient relations as well as attempts to distance themselves from the practices of traditional institutions. When we describe particular communities we shall use the nomenclature of the community, for example, 'co-workers' and 'children' at the Camphill communities. When we are embarking on more general analyses we shall use the term 'resident', which, though not equally applicable to each of our communities, allows us to avoid the clumsy neologism 'patient/resident'. Where the staff-resident divide is irrelevant to the issue at hand we shall use the term 'community members'.

Chapter 1

The historical development of therapeutic community approaches

The aim of this chapter is to provide a fairly short historical account of the development of therapeutic community techniques, which will offer a wider context for our own work and be of some interest to readers who may be unfamiliar with the many different branches of the therapeutic communities movement. In some ways our account here will be unavoidably deficient: we are not professional historians and have not used original sources. Moreover, we are aware that good short histories of some types of therapeutic communities already exist, for example, Manning's account, published in 1976, of the development of communities in residential psychiatric units, written from a sociology of science perspective. Two more general historical surveys can also be recommended: the first part of David Kennard's recent introductory text on therapeutic communities (Kennard, 1983); and the chapter on therapeutic communities in Whiteley and Gordon (1979), although both studies deal only briefly with certain types of therapeutic communities (such as the Camphill communities) with which we will be concerned in this book. To repeat, our purpose here is less to capture every nuance in the development of therapeutic community approaches than to provide a wide historical context against which our own work can be placed.

Foster family communities

The oldest variety of community is the 'foster family' community, exemplified in our study by Parkneuk. The best known of these communities, Geel in Flanders, can trace its origins back to the Middle Ages; since at least 1250, and well prior to the establishment of Europe's first psychiatric hospital in Valencia, the townspeople of

Geel have been opening their doors to mentally afflicted pilgrims who came to worship at the local shrine of St Dymphna (Roosens, 1979).

Over the centuries the practice of boarding pilgrims in the town slowly changed from temporary makeshifts to permanent arrangements negotiated between the individual families in the town and the kin of the boarders, and overseen by the local church canons. In 1850 the supervision of boarding arrangements was taken over by the Belgian state and in 1862 an in-patient facility (the 'Kolonie') was set up to oversee the boarding arrangements and to provide a small number of beds, both for the observation of new would-be boarders, and for the temporary treatment of boarders whom the foster families found unmanageable. Although the numbers of families in Geel willing to admit boarders has fallen steadily since the last war, the 30000 people of Geel still took in 1300 boarders in 1975, which amounted to 5.8 per cent of the total population in Belgian psychiatric institutions (Roosens, 1979). So Geel is the largest, as well as the oldest, therapeutic community in the world.

Geel tends to be used by the state as a dumping ground for chronic cases with a long history of institutionalisation; the predominant diagnosis is schizophrenia. The effectiveness of the Geel regime is difficult to assess. Roosens points out that around 30 of the 1300 boarders are discharged per annum because of significant improvement, which is not bad for a predominantly 'chronic' patient population (Roosens, p. 185). Srole (1977) cites an unpublished paper by Pierloot, reporting on the follow-up of 64 patients transferred from the Kortenberg Hospital to Geel families. The hospital considered that prospects for further clinical improvement in these cases was 'very limited'. On follow-up, 2 of the 64 patients had died and 4 had returned to their natural families; 9 patients had been rehospitalised (4 because they were French-speaking and had difficulties with the native Flemish of the Geelians); the remaining 49 were 'relatively well integrated' and more than 80 per cent of them showed enhanced 'social functioning' (Srole, pp. 119–20). Roosens observed that nearly all the Geel boarders 'like it better there than in the institution or institutions from which they came. The greatest threat hanging over them is another period of confinement "inside".' (Roosens, p. 185).

The host families of Geel are remunerated by the state. The fees are universally agreed to be too low, particularly when set against the cost of hospital care, but it is the fees which provide the main motivation for Geelians to take in a patient. Historically, many of the townspeople possessed small agricultural holdings (similar to Scottish Highland 'crofts') which were worked part-time and provided enough for their own needs with a small surplus for market; the foster families of Geel came predominantly from this group of poor crofters, and their boarders found occupation in domestic and agricultural work about the croft. Part of the reason for the decline in the numbers is undoubtedly the increasing affluence of the townspeople, along with the decreasing proportion of the population involved in agriculture. Despite the inadequate fees paid to host families, many still find it economically worthwhile to take in boarders since fees are remitted twice a year and so take on the character of a nest egg which can be set aside for, say, house purchase or a child's university education.

Despite the fact that the economic value of the boarders' labour has declined (in the past it was allegedly commonplace for families to bribe the Kolonie nurse in order to be allocated a good worker), for a minority of families the boarders' labour remains crucially important. The Kolonie staff now provides additional activities for boarders in the form of work therapy, sports clubs, and outings, which supplement boarders' activities with host families.

Inevitably, the Geel system is open to allegations of exploitation of the boarders, though local public opinion seems a strong check on such abuses; removal by the Kolonie of a boarder is seen as a great disgrace and host families also take a keen interest in the weight gain of boarders, revealed at the regular medical examinations, since this is taken as an indication of good treatment! Moreover, although the initial motivation for taking a boarder may be economic, the motivation for keeping a boarder who has been adopted into the family circle transcends economics. It is normal, for example, for grown-up children to take over responsibility for a patient who was boarded with their parents.

Similar systems to that of Geel are found in a number of European countries. The family care colony at Beilen in Holland was set up in the 1920s in imitation of Geel, where many Dutch patients were formerly boarded. At Beilen relatively more neurotic patients were boarded than at Geel (Wing, 1957). In Norway the boarding out of patients was common throughout the country in the 1950s as a response to the overcrowding of psychiatric hospitals, but boarders were particularly concentrated in the Lier Valley, where at the time of Wing's visit 1000 of the population of 14000 were boarders (Wing,

1957). In recent years the growth of radical community psychiatry in Italy has led to many somewhat similar experiments there, although the Geel system has probably not had a direct influence on these developments.

Although the research of Srole and his colleagues in Geel (Srole, 1977) has stimulated interest in foster communities among American psychiatrists, similar interest has largely been lacking in Britain. Family care has never been a feature of English psychiatry except in the form of guardianship, although in Scotland the literal 'farming out' of psychiatric patients was widespread up to the First World War (for a fictional account of these boarders in a Scottish rural community, see Lewis Grassic Gibbon's classic *Sunset Song, passim*). In Britain the main impetus towards foster family care has come from social workers. Experiments such as that of the Kent Social Services Department in a paid fostering scheme for children have been extended to other areas of the country and other client groups, most notably the frail elderly, and the mentally handicapped. However, the social work departments have not attempted to concentrate their efforts on recruiting host families in particular localities where the families can benefit from mutual support, and, in some departments at least, social workers have attempted to screen out applicant families whom they judge to have a mainly financial motivation!

By and large, we must turn to private charitable initiatives if we wish to find British examples of foster family communities, either in the sense of geographical localities or of large communal households. The Camphill movement is best known for its residential schools for mentally handicapped and disturbed children; however, in addition to these schools there are also a number of centres where handicapped and disturbed adults live alongside Camphill co-workers in a naturalistic, if not natural, domestic environment. In Stourbridge, Worcestershire, for example, three houses have been purchased in the town to enable a small number of handicapped adults and co-workers to live as normal a life as possible in an urban setting – adults work in the town and attend a variety of local social functions. Contrastingly, there are a number of Camphill village estates, like Newton Dee in Aberdeenshire and Grange-Oakland in Gloucestershire, where quite large numbers of handicapped adults and co-workers form their own more self-reliant communities in a variety of rural settings. Whereas in the Stourbridge homes an attempt is made to maximise the involvement of the adults in the normal life of the town, within the village estates the attempt is rather more to form communities in their own right with adults working the land, producing a variety of craft goods and attending their own social functions.

Similar attempts to enable handicapped adults to live naturalistic lives of economic and social independence include the now defunct Kingsway Community (see Rigby, 1974) and the Cyrenians' farm outside Edinburgh.

A number of ex-Camphill co-workers have undertaken fostering after their departure from Camphill communities. In some instances couples have simply accepted children from Camphill communities in school holidays where the children have no natural parents to return to. In other instances ex-Camphill couples have fostered children with whom they formerly lived at Camphill once those children have passed school age. Again, household economics is an important motivation: the fees the couples receive from the child's local authority (or, more rarely, the natural parents) enable them to pursue occupations in arts and crafts, or horticulture, which would otherwise be financially nonviable. Sometimes these ex-Camphill co-workers have formed small communities of their own, where co-workers willing to share their lives with their disturbed and handicapped boarders have found that the boarders' fees provide a financial cushion which furnishes the necessities for simple communal living and allows co-workers and boarders alike the freedom to pursue a developing interest in, say, handloom weaving, or bee-keeping, or furniture-making. 'Parkneuk', one of our study settings, is such a community. An analogous initiative in the state sector is the Cardiff Scheme, in which university students are provided with free accommodation in group homes for the mentally handicapped.

Leaving aside Geel's seven-hundred-year history, it is sometimes claimed that therapeutic communities began with the social experiments of Pinel in Paris asylums and of Tuke at the Quaker 'Retreat' in York in the late eighteenth and early nineteenth century. This is a bit of a fiction. Although there certainly are parallels between Tuke's 'moral treatment' regime at The Retreat and the regimes in modern hospital communities, there was no continuity of practice between Tuke's work in the 1820s and the first modern hospital community at Northfield Military Hospital in the 1940s; as the nineteenth century progressed, and the mental hospitals swelled enormously in size, Tuke's work was largely forgotten and the asylums entered on their long custodial sleep (Scull, 1979; Kennard, 1983).

Homer Lane and planned environment therapy

A more genealogically accurate candidate for the position of father of the movement (at least in the English-speaking world) is that charismatic and eccentric figure, Homer Lane (1875–1925). Lane was a New England woodwork teacher who developed an interest in, and an extraordinary ascendancy over, delinquent boys; he was appointed superintendent of the Detroit Playgrounds and then, in 1907, took up the post of superintendent at a residential institution for juvenile offenders that was eventually to be known as 'The Boys' Republic' (Wills, 1964).

Lane moved the institution from Detroit to a 70-acre farm 20 miles outside the city. His management committee wanted to have the house and outbuildings thoroughly cleaned before the new inhabitants took up residence, but Lane would have none of this. He believed that the boys would value the house more highly if they cleaned it themselves. And they did (Wills, 1964, p. 77). He and the boys set about planning and erecting another building: they dug the foundations, cast the blocks and mixed the concrete. Their work remains today the central building of The Boys' Republic (Wills, 1964, p. 78). An elaborate constitution was inaugurated, modelled on the US Constitution: the superintendent was Chief Justice of the Court and also had a right of veto over government decisions, but this veto could be overturned by a two-thirds majority of the legislative assembly, which included all citizens over ten years of age (Wills, 1964, p. 82). Lane sought to replace close supervision and an emphasis on successful task-performance by a group ideal of collective and individual responsibility for behaviour. By personal influence and example he led boys to make the right choices, but by allowing free choice and self-expression he aimed to develop latent capabilities.

Lane's regime seems to have been a great success, and his own charm and gift of public relations ensured that the success did not go unremarked. A stream of visitors, including the eminent sociologist Professor Charles Cooley and an influential Englishman, George Montagu, the future ninth Earl of Sandwich, all sang the praises of Lane's Republic. But in 1912 Lane was forced to resign: his management committee, already somewhat exasperated by Lane's financial irresponsibility, could not stomach his open affair with a woman teacher at the Republic (Wills, 1964, pp. 120–1).

In 1913 the Montagu connection saw Lane appointed as first superintendent of the Little Commonwealth, established in converted farm buildings on the Earl of Sandwich's estates in Dorset (Wills, 1964, pp. 129–30). In the interval Lane appears to have been reading Pestalozzi, and at The Little Commonwealth he laid greater stress on the influence of affectionate relations than he had at The Boys' Republic, and there was less stress on the punishment of transgressions (Wills, 1964, p. 137); the daily round and the machinery of government remained much the same. The Little Commonwealth took girls as well as boys, and not just delinquents, but also toddlers as young as two under the auspices of the Montessori Society. Through conversion and new building the Little Commonwealth eventually comprised four cottages for living accommodation (the younger children in a separate cottage), a school, an executive block and a workshop. Remarkably, the then Home Office Inspector certified this revolutionary establishment as a reformatory, so that local authorities were authorised to fund the Commonwealth by paying the childrens' fees.

This climate of government patronage was not maintained, however. Home Office certification of the Commonwealth was withdrawn following an inquiry into allegations of sexual improprieties made against Lane by some of the girls. The findings of the inquiry were not made public but Wills, Lane's biographer, believed that the allegations were merely a pretext for withdrawing support from a regime with which officials were not in sympathy, the original certifying inspector having died in the interim. It is undeniable that Lane had behaved most imprudently in, for example, being served early morning coffee in his bedroom by the girls. However, Wills's inference seems the correct one in view of the fact that the Home Office made no attempt to remove the girls concerned from Lane's care after the inquiry (Wills, 1964, pp. 186–95).

The withdrawal of certification was a disastrous blow to the Commonwealth's finances, and although the management committee had complete confidence in Lane they were forced to close the Commonwealth in 1918. Lane then set up in practice as a psychotherapist (not being medically qualified, he took 'pupils', for 'instruction'). His pupils included the great and the good – a future viceroy of India, a future cabinet minister, and the like. Scandal struck again. Lane (still an American citizen and therefore an alien) was charged with failing to register his change of address with the police. Instead of a forty-shilling fine, Lane found himself remanded in custody awaiting possible deportation as an undesirable alien because of his acceptance of large financial gifts from a psychotic young woman who was one of his pupils. The proceedings became a nine day wonder. Letters from Lane's files implying that he had indulged in adulterous affairs with some of his pupils were read out in court. Bishops and peers mustered in Lane's defence, and finally a backstage deal was struck which left the deportation order unsigned so long as Lane left the country voluntarily.

Worn down by the strain, Lane died in Paris some five months later. W. H. Auden, for one, did not believe pneumonia to be the real culprit:

> Lawrence was brought down by Smuthounds, Blake went dotty as he
> sang,
> Homer Lane was killed in action by the Twickenham Baptist Gang.

But Lane is more than a 50-year-old cause célèbre; his influence on the therapeutic communities movement has been profound. His lectures and addresses were collected and published posthumously and one of his helpers wrote a book about the Little Commonwealth (Bazeley, 1928). Lane's main influcncc, though, has been through the work of his associates. David Wills, Lane's biographer, both worked and wrote extensively in the field of residential care for maladjusted children – see his account of Hawkspur Camp, a quaker workcamp for maladjusted youths (Wills, 1941); his account of Reynolds House, a residential community for twelve maladjusted youths (Wills, 1970); and his more general work, *Spare the Child* (Wills, 1971). Wills acknowledged that 'Homer Lane was the root and inspiration of all our work at Hawkspur Camp' (Wills, 1941, p. 137) and that 'in the new schools for maladjusted children ... Lane's influence is clearly to be seen' (Wills, 1964, p. 139).

A. S. Neill, of Summerhill fame, was on the point of joining the staff of the Little Commonwealth when the Home Office sank it. Neill became a 'pupil' of Lane's when he set up as a psychotherapist and was an intimate of Lane's family circle. The personal and intellectual influence of Lane on Neill's life and work was enormous: 'Neill's two years as pupil of Lane gave him both the momentum and the inspiration to clarify his goal, which was now to work with children "the Little Commonwealth way".' (Croall, 1983, p. 96)

Through the influence of successors like Wills and Neill, Lane's approach has spread abroad and into different treatment settings, but official endorsement remains problematic (hardly surprisingly in view of Lane's relations with the Home Office!). The development of therapeutic community methods in List D Schools for juvenile offenders was set back by the Godfrey Thomson Unit study of Loaningdale Approved School, which showed that reconviction rates for ex-Loaningdale boys were no lower than reconviction rates for the other Scottish approved schools (McMichael, 1972, p. 93), and Loaningdale was subsequently closed. As regards adult penal institutions, H. M. Prison at Grendon (England) and the Barlinnie Special Unit (Scotland) are therapeutic communities of long standing but they have not led to changes in the remainder of the penal system. As we shall see in relation to other types of therapeutic community, it is a common pattern for therapeutic community methods to be advocated enthusiastically as a worthwhile approach to the care and/or treatment of some disadvantaged or disabled group, only for this initiative to ossify at the point where a few experimental institutions have been introduced. These experimental communities usually persist (despite recurrent criticism and occasional scandals), sustained by the enthusiasm of their members and the vulnerability of officialdom to determined lobbying, but only rarely do they lead to generalised changes in service provision (Manning, 1976a). Instead, the tendency is for them to become onlookers while new generations of innovators attempt to capture the very services that the earlier community advocates had hoped to secure. It is beyond the scope of this survey to suggest reasons why this should be so, but it is impossible not to feel some sympathy for, say, advocates of therapeutic communities in the penal services as they contemplate the current faddish growth of 'short, sharp shock' methods.

The Camphill movement

Chronologically, the next development in the growth of therapeutic communities was the foundation of the Camphill movement in 1938 by the Viennese general practitioner Karl Konig. It was Konig's belief that, in addition to providing care for handicapped children in individual households, what was necessary was to create a new social, spiritual, and economic setting within which they could live and develop as equals – a setting that was described, at that time, as a 'therapeutic state of community' (Weihs, 1965). As Konig envisaged the community, it was to be based on ideas and principles derived from the work of the Austrian philosopher and mystic Rudolf Steiner. Before his death in 1925, Steiner had built upon his own spiritual experiences to elaborate a system of ideas known as Anthroposophy, which sought to depict humans as spiritual beings and human development as a process of incarnation from the spirit world. In addition to applying these schemes to such diverse fields as agriculture, architecture and education, Steiner had also developed a long-term interest in the development of handicapped children. As a young man, Steiner had been given responsibility for the education of an apparently subnormal, hydrocephalic child, regarded by his previous tutors as ineducable. Through hours of painstaking preparation, however, Steiner devised a curriculum which addressed the child's many difficulties and which, through their subsequent work together, enabled the boy to enter university and qualify as a medical practitioner (Steiner, 1928, pp. 71–7).

Towards the end of his life Steiner delivered a short lecture course on curative education (*Heilpaedagogik*) in which he argued that characteristic patterns of behaviour in handicapped and disturbed children could often be traced to imbalances occurring in the process whereby spiritual forces entered into and worked upon the physical body. Bed-wetting and epileptic fits were just two examples which he cited as indicative of particular imbalances occurring in the process of incarnation from the spirit world to the physical world. In close collaboration with others Steiner also sought to devise various remedies for the reparation of such imbalances. Curative eurythmy was one such therapy. Based upon specific movement exercises, it was designed to facilitate the correct incarnation of spirit forces into the child. Parenthetically, it is worth adding here that there is no necessary clash between Steiner's ideas and allopathic medicine since Steiner's ideas were oriented towards caring for, say, the child with Down's Syndrome rather than with providing an alternative and conflicting explanation of the genetic basis of the syndrome itself.

Although Konig sought to employ Steiner's ideas in creating a community environment for the handicapped child, before much could be done in this vein Austria was overrun by the Nazis and he and his colleagues had to flee to Scotland. There too, however, the small group was beset with difficulties. Soon after their arrival all male members of the group were interned as enemy aliens and the creation of what was to be the new 'therapeutic state of community' was left to the remaining few women. Fortunately, Steiner's ideas had already secured a small audience in Britain and with the help of the influential W. F. Macmillan, who was at that time looking for a place where his own handicapped son could be cared for, the group was able to purchase a small estate near Aberdeen.

Steiner's ideas did not provide a simple blueprint for practice in the new community, rather his ideas were adapted to fit the new circumstances. The school curriculum was developed from that devised by Steiner for the normal child. Similarly, in the early days a good deal of authority was vested in the post of medical superintendent. Subsequently, the attempt was made to create a new social order within the community based upon what Steiner had described as 'the threefold social order': fraternity in the economic life of the community, equality in the need for mutual cooperation between community members, and liberty in the need for individual privacy within the community.

The community differed physically as well as socially from its surrounding environment, in that it used Steiner's ideas on architecture and agriculture – and even today one searches Camphill in vain for a television set.

The growth of the community was slow in the beginning, though gradually other houses were added to the original buildings. In 1945, and again with the help of the Macmillan family, a nearby village estate (Newton Dee) was purchased, originally with the intention of providing a home for delinquent boys, though subsequently being used for sheltered workshops and long-term accommodation for many of the Camphill 'graduates'. Eventually the example of Camphill led anthroposophists to establish similar centres elsewhere in Britain and abroad, particularly in the countries of northern Europe.

By the time of Konig's death in 1966 expansion had become rapid. Most of the income of the communities came from fees from the children's local authorities. Donations and bequests from anthroposophists, parents and sympathisers provided capital for new buildings and new communities. Some local authorities refused to consider Camphill placements while they had places in their special schools for the mentally handicapped, but other authorities were impressed by the fact that the level of fees compared favourably with the total costs of places at their special schools, and by the fact that the Camphill communities were able to provide very high carer-to-children ratios so that standards of care were self-evidently high. Waiting lists lengthened. The bulk of the co-workers comprised a kind of international peace corps of young people of all religions and none, many of whom had been educated in Waldorf Schools, who came to serve as co-workers for one or two years. Some communities found themselves having to operate a waiting list for co-workers as well as children.

The communities began to consider expanding their services to cover different disabilities and handicaps. The opening of Newton Dee for adults has already been mentioned. Experiments were also begun with new therapies, for example, music and drama therapy, coloured light therapy, and, perhaps most important of all, the interactive therapeutic effects of different disabilities, particularly those associated with combining Down's Syndrome and autistic children in the same house or dormitory, were explored. Most recently a community has been opened caring for the infirm elderly.

Today the original Camphill Rudolf Steiner Schools community is the titular head of a Camphill movement spread across 17 countries. Although no accurate census of Camphill and its offshoots exists, it has been estimated that worldwide there are approximately 8000 individuals (carers and cared for) resident within Camphill centres. Camphill, then, is undoubtedly one of the most populous of all the different types of therapeutic communities currently in existence.

Nevertheless, there is some uncertainty as to whether previous growth will be maintained: the readiness of the authorities in Britain to meet fees has inevitably been affected by central government cutbacks. Also, the future eligibility of the communities to receive fees will depend upon government recognition of the training courses for Camphill co-workers. Despite these difficulties, senior members of the movement continue to endorse the Utopian vision of the founders, who believed that curative education would grow to the point where it transformed the wider society from within.

The growth of the Camphill movement has been almost silent and unremarked. Only a relatively small number of psychiatrists and social workers have a working knowledge of practice in the Steiner communities, and references to Camphill in professional journals are almost non-existent. Even among fellow therapeutic community practitioners knowledge of Camphill is very limited, although Newton Dee village has joined the Association of Therapeutic

Communities. We hope that our comparative survey will help to go some way towards remedying this deficiency.

The Camphill movement is not unique; other therapeutic communities have been established quite independently since the war, following similar communal principles and motivated by similar Utopian religious impulses. For example, there are the catholic L'Arche communities first established by the French Canadian Jean Vanier in 1964 to provide permanent homes for the mentally handicapped. L'Arche communities are now spread throughout the French-speaking world and are also found in America, England, Scotland, Denmark and India. L'Arche provides sheltered workshops and some residents live at L'Arche and work outside the community. There is no formal therapeutic intervention – therapy is held to consist in the affectionate relations between the handicapped and their 'assistants' as they share their social, working, and spiritual lives. In the L'Arche community reported on by Clarke, a weekly meeting chaired by a local psychiatrist helped the assistants to maintain a reflective (but not detached) attitude to their work (Clarke, 1974, pp. 101–9).

Hospital communities

The next development which follows chronologically from the Camphill movement is the upheaval in institutional psychiatry occasioned by the Second World War and the subsequent establishment of therapeutic communities within psychiatric hospitals. As we mentioned at the outset, this is a development that has been particularly well documented elsewhere (e.g. Manning, 1976a) and we will do little more than summarise these works here.

Hospital psychiatry between the wars was little different from that of the Victorian era. The work of Freud and later academic innovators like Sullivan and Lewin had done nothing to alter the dreary custodial regimes of the great asylums. The war created a great demand for trained psychiatrists and offered junior personnel the chance to develop new techniques in senior positions. Two centres of innovation can be distinguished where therapeutic community methods were developed independently and contemporaneously. At the Northfield Military Hospital a group from the Tavistock Clinic attempted to treat neuroses by improving social relationships in the hospital and devolving administrative functions

(Main, 1946). One of this group, Tom Main, applied these principles to peace-time hospital psychiatry on his appointment as medical superintendent at Cassel Hospital in 1947.

At Cassel Hospital, Main and his colleagues have pursued an independent (and unique) line of development which entailed a sharp distinction between the roles of psychiatrist and psychiatric nurses. The nurses interacted with the (neurotic) patients as 'co-citizens' in the performance of a programme of maintenance and cleaning tasks. The psychiatrists practised psychoanalytically-orientated individual and group psychotherapy. As Kennard puts it, 'in effect there was a quite deliberate separation between the "outer" world of social roles, work tasks and current relationships, and the "inner" world of private fantasy and feelings.' (Kennard, 1983, p. 54).

The other centre of innovation was the Effort Syndrome Unit led by Maxwell Jones at Mill Hill School. The unit was devoted to the treatment of patients who were neurotically anxious about possible heart disease. Jones began a series of didactic lectures to patients on the psychosomatic basis of their heart pains; the lectures evolved into an open discussion format and Jones recognised the importance of the role of senior patients in producing insight into their condition among junior patients. Jones was led to attempting to reproduce in the social life of the ward the same social situations that his patients had faced in life outside. He continued his experiments with discharged prisoners-of-war; subsequently the Ministry of Labour gave him charge of the Belmont Industrial Neurosis Unit (now Henderson Hospital), initially for the rehabilitation of neurotic unemployables, and finally for the treatment of personality disorders. Jones produced a steady stream of books and articles from the Belmont unit, which was also the topic of a pioneering study by the American anthropologist Robert Rapoport (1960). Rapoport's description of the Belmont unit eventually became a sort of textbook of hospital therapeutic community practice.

Alert readers will already have discerned a pattern here – Lane and the Little Commonwealth, Konig and the Camphill movement, Jones and the hospital communities. We are not peddling a 'great man' theory of history; the prominence of these personalities in our story simply reflects the importance of charismatic leadership in the early stages of development of any innovatory service. Certainly, Jones performed this charismatic function for the hospital communities. A flood of influential visitors passed through the Belmont unit; a number were inspired by Jones and his unit to attempt to set up similar communities. Such was the pivotal importance of Jones's leadership that a WHO report (1953) doubted whether Jones's methods would have met with the same success under different leadership – a judgment that had earlier been made of Homer Lane's Boys' Republic.

However, the process of the diffusion of the innovation was also a process of dilution. The term 'therapeutic community' became a buzz-word like 'teamwork' or 'community care'. Moreover, some of the by-products of Jones's methods, such as respect for the patients' individuality and the organisation of a daily programme of patient activities, accorded well with the new conditions of psychiatric hospitals in the 1950s, where the use of the new tranquillising drugs had reduced the need for custodial care and the great majority of new admissions were voluntary. Not surprisingly, then, it became commonplace for hospital psychiatrists to claim their regimes to be therapeutic communities, despite the fact that these regimes bore only superficial resemblances to the pioneer communities of Jones and Main: democracy applied to the running of the social clubs, not to patient involvement in ward government. This watering down of Jones's methods and the resultant definitional confusion led Clark (1965) to distinguish between the 'therapeutic community proper' (à la Jones) and the 'therapeutic community approach'.

Twelve years later Clark reviewed the position and concluded that his earlier distinction was no longer a necessary one (Clark, 1977). The liberalisation of hospital regimes implicit in the 'therapeutic community approach' was now almost universal, but these regimes were less likely to claim the title of 'therapeutic community' since the term was no longer in vogue. Some of the British therapeutic communities proper were still extant (Clark enumerated six in England), but in America, where Jones's work had found many enthusiastic imitators, those communities had 'gone like the hula-hoop' (Clark, 1977, p. 555) and the very term 'therapeutic community' had changed its signification to the more recently developed 'concept houses' for the treatment of addiction. In some European countries (notably the Netherlands) hospital communities were widely established, but elsewhere – France, for example (Herzlich, 1976) – reform efforts were concentrated on the development of community alternatives to psychiatric hospitals rather than the transformation of hospital practice. In Germany the links between therapeutic community practice and political radicalism led to a much-publicised police raid on a community and the forcible dispersal of the patients; other German communities were condemned by association.

The hospital communities had suffered from an intellectual seachange in institutional psychiatry. It would be difficult to try and identify any single factor responsible for that change: it is likely that the relative demise of hospital-based communities was the result of a number of factors operating in concert. The development of new pharmacological treatments excited and attracted a new generation of psychiatrists, and while visitors still flocked to the old Belmont unit (now renamed the Henderson Hospital) most of them were social workers and probation officers rather than psychiatrists and nurses (Manning, 1976a). A number of articles critical of therapeutic communities were published in academic journals (e.g. Zeitlyn, 1967; Raskin, 1971). There was some confusion over those diagnostic groups for whom therapeutic community methods were most appropriate. In earlier days, psychiatrists had implemented Jones's approach across a broad range of diagnostic labels, and Jones himself (having moved to Dingleton Hospital in the Scottish Borders) was applying his work to psychogeriatrics (Jones, 1982). But a follow-up study of patients from the Littlemore Hospital in Oxford found therapeutic community methods to be of no more value than traditional methods in the treatment of schizophrenia (Letemendia et al., 1967). These findings were disputed by another follow-up study of schizophrenic patients conducted by Myers and Clark (1972), but increasingly hospital psychiatrists practising in therapeutic communities began to follow Martin (1972) in concentrating their efforts on chronic neurotic patients.

The shift in emphasis in British psychiatry from hospital to community psychiatry need not have been deleterious to the therapeutic communities. At Dingleton, Jones had been a pioneer of community psychiatry methods to prevent in-patient admission for acute mental breakdown (Morrice, 1966; Jones, 1968, 1982), and many felt that those psychiatric day hospitals being set up in the 1960s would be ideally suited to therapeutic community methods. Yet in the event very few of the day hospitals outside London were organised as therapeutic communities: in Scotland, for example, only Aberdeen's Ross Clinic day hospital was organised along therapeutic community lines (Morrice, 1973).

Government policy envisages the main area of institutional growth in psychiatric services to be the increased provision of day care centres under the auspices of local authority social services departments. These centres could in principle be run along therapeutic community lines, as is demonstrated by the St Luke's project (involving three day care centres) in the London borough of Kensington and Chelsea (Blake, 1977). However, the St Luke's Project has not been extensively imitated.

The future of the hospital communities is unclear. On the one hand, the continuing vigour of the hospital communities is evidenced by the fact that it was the staff of these communities who founded the Association of Therapeutic Communities, which has become an important forum for the discussion of innovation and research. Further, there is scope for a number of collaborative ventures between psychiatrists and social services departments to set up local day care centres run as therapeutic communities and this may indicate a line of future development. And finally, recent attempts to shut down therapeutic communities such as the Paddington Day Hospital and the Henderson Hospital have been sharply contested.

On the other hand, a number of commentators and practitioners can be heard arguing that psychiatric hospitals are not suitable host institutions for therapeutic communities, that too much staff energy must be diverted from patient care to defending the community from attacks from unsympathetic colleagues and administrators (e.g. Cooper, 1967; Myers, 1979; Hoffman and Singer, 1977). And if it is acknowledged that attempts to shut down communities have been contested, sometimes successfully, it must also be recognised that most of the hospital communities that have disappeared in recent years have done so as a result of the death, departure, or retirement of the consultant in charge: frequently, the new appointee has no interest in therapeutic community methods and junior staff lose heart or take up posts elsewhere.

The concept house

The next chronological development in the therapeutic communities movement was the foundation of the Synanon community in California in 1958. Again, there is a charismatic leader, Chuck Dederich, an ex-alcoholic and campaigner for Alcoholics Anonymous who started Synanon for the treatment of drug addicts in his flat with his 33-dollar unemployment cheque (Ofshe et al., 1974). Ten years later Synanon had over 1200 resident members in communities from New York to Puerto Rico and assets worth 6 million dollars (Kanter, 1972).

Although the structure and practices of Synanon, and of subsequent 'concept houses' which followed it, owed much to Dederich's experiences in AA, various commentators have also pointed out strong parallels with religious sects: 'the total dedication to the moral and spiritual improvement of members; the use of public confession and mutual criticism; the elimination of privacy; the hierarchy of authority based on moral and spiritual superiority; the procedures for the mortification of deviants and for periodically generating states of ecstatic love and joy within the group' (Sugarman, 1975, p. 141). We might also mention the belief by some adherents that Dederich is God, Jesus, or (more mildly) a modern Socrates (quoted in Kanter, 1972), and the reiteration at every morning meeting of the Synanon prayer ('Please let me first and always examine myself. Let me be honest and truthful...'). There is also the fact that senior members of the community are themselves converts, ex-addicts who have seen the light in Synanon. In view of all this it was perhaps not surprising that in 1975 – seventeen years after its foundation – Synanon should indeed proclaim itself as a religion.

In its early days the sectarian character of Synanon, its unconventional treatment approach, and the disreputable character of its clientele all brought a good deal of publicity. The ultra-conservative citizens of Santa Monica secured a conviction against Dederich for violating the city's house zoning laws. A film, *The House on the Beach*, described the original Synanon house. Newspaper stories were legion. The socially prominent lent their support or denounced the approach as 'brainwashing' and Dederich as a 'megalomaniac' (quoted in Kanter, 1972). All this attention provided publicity for Synanon's claim to be the only successful treatment programme for addicts. The claim was a contentious one: certainly, the Synanon programme was highly effective for ex-addicts who successfully graduated from the community, but the majority of entrants did not graduate – they dropped out. Of the 263 addicts admitted to Synanon between May 1958 and May 1961, 190 (72%) left against the advice of Synanon staff, 59% of these drop-outs occurred in the first month of their residence and 90% within the first three months (Volkman and Cressey, 1963). The inclusion of this drop-out population dramatically reduces Synanon's success rate, but it is arguable that the approach was still more effective than the available alternatives. According to Volkman and Cressey (1963), of the total number of Synanon enrolees up to August 1962, 108 (29%)

were known to be off drugs, and of the 215 that had remained in Synanon at that period for more than one month, 103 (48%) were known to be off drugs at the time the study was conducted. Shelly compared success rates (no convictions and gainful employment) for a group from a similar community (Daytop Village) with a control group on probation: the Daytop success rate (drop-outs included) was 35%, for the controls on probation the success rate was only 4% (cited in Sugarman, 1974, pp. 6–7). As we shall argue elsewhere however, figures from such evaluative studies have to be treated with considerable caution: those entering Daytop may have been more motivated than the controls to remain drug-free.

Synanon's claim of treatment effectiveness and its innovative image encouraged a host of imitative communities in America in the 1960s as the authorities tried to respond to the rising tide of heroin addiction in American cities; Kanter writes of 'hundreds' of concept houses (so called because they followed the Synanon 'concept') – certainly over a hundred were established. The most prominent of these new concept houses were the eleven Phoenix houses treating around 1000 people (Rosenthal, 1980). In 1968 three ex-addict graduates of the Phoenix House programme in New York were employed by the London Boroughs Association to set up a London concept house. The first Dutch concept house was established by Kooyman, a psychiatrist, at The Hague in 1971.

Unlike its imitators, Synanon had always remained independent of government and municipal financial support and in 1968 Dederich felt able to renounce any rehabilitative function: Synanon henceforth was to be a fully fledged Utopian social movement which entrants joined for life, with its own businesses, where non-addict 'lifestylers' were encouraged to join the communities; Synanon was to transform society by wholesale conversion to the Synanon Way (Kanter, 1972).

The current position of the concept houses is uncertain. In Britain there are now five such houses (with their own Association of Concept-Based Therapeutic Communities), the best known of which is the Ley Community in Oxford, which has been well described by Kennard (1983, pp. 64–84). The period of treatment in such communities is lengthy (typically eighteen months to two years), and therefore expensive. The government has expressed a preference for cheaper, non-residential, treatment options. In Holland, similar criticism has led concept houses and associated halfway houses to revise downwards the expected length of stay in each of the institutions to periods of six months. One of the Dutch houses has followed a similar path to Synanon and become a Bagwan community (following the teachings of Bagwan Shri Rajneesh). With a slow-down in the expansion of concept houses it has been suggested that relapses may become more prevalent among graduates, since in the past many have found employment in new concept houses where they are sustained in their abstinence and newly-learned behaviour patterns.

Halfway house communities

The origins of halfway house therapeutic communities are a matter for debate. Halfway houses, as institutions to bridge the gap between the psychiatric hospital and the wider community, have been around for over a century (the Mental After-Care Association was founded in 1879), but their history as institutions where everyday activities and relationships are self-consciously redefined for a therapeutic purpose is rather shorter. Spring Lake Ranch in Vermont was established in 1932 and has been described by some as a halfway house; in our nomenclature it might be described more accurately as a foster family care therapeutic community, since it is communally organised with naturalistic living and working relationships, and no formally therapeutic groups or meetings (Wells, 1980). A less controversial candidate for the accolade of original halfway house therapeutic community would be the Richmond Fellowship.

The Fellowship was started up in 1959 by a young Dutch theology student, Elly Jansen, in a rented house in suburban London, as a community for ex-psychiatric hospital patients (Jansen, 1970, 1980a, 1980b). In the same year the Mental Health Act was passed, giving local authorities the power to substitute residential community care for hospital care. The founding of the Fellowship thus coincided with official recognition that new institutional forms were required to cater for the flood of psychiatric patients now being discharged from the hospitals, but often with no families able or willing to receive them and with continuing problems, not least so-called 'institutional neuroses' (Barton, 1959). Despite the unwillingness of some local authorities to fund places in Fellowship houses, the growth of the Fellowship (under Elly Jansen's charismatic directorship) was rapid. Twenty-five years later the Fellowship had 45 communities in Britain (catering for 726 residents) and had established communities in America, Australia, New Zealand, and Austria (Jansen, 1984).

In the interim the Fellowship had broadened its remit from ex-psychiatric patients: two houses were set up for ex-alcoholics, one for ex-drug addicts, one for the mentally handicapped, and (most importantly) ten houses were set up for disturbed and maladjusted adolescents. The increasing involvement of the Fellowship with an adolescent client group may be linked to the realisation by funding agencies that the supposed insecurities of adolescence and difficulties of family relationships self-evidently demand residential care (as opposed to day care) facilities.

It will be appreciated that these different client groups preclude any single organisational format within the Fellowship houses, but even between similarly circumstanced communities the Fellowship houses show a mix of therapeutic community approaches, with some communities employing permissive regimes reminiscent of the Maxwell Jones-type hospital communities, and others employing a more hierarchical regime similar to (but less punitive than) the concept houses. In recent years the Fellowship has been a pioneer in therapeutic community settings of the 'psycho-education' approach developed in Canada: adolescent behavioural and personality problems are seen as arising from faulty 'epigenetic' development. Treatment involves the very detailed individual programming of every child's every activity, so that the adolescent is 're-educated' by reproducing the various phases of their child development in a manner that is no longer faulty and cumulatively damaging (Gauthier, 1980). There are clearly logistical difficulties in achieving a high degree of staff planning in residential settings which naturally demand long hours of staff-resident contact, but it is too early to comment on the success of a psycho-education approach in adolescent therapeutic communities – the Fellowship's St Nicholas House, specifically designed as a psycho-education community, was only opened in 1981.

All the Fellowship houses employ a warden, deputy warden and other care staff (some of whom are normally residential), working on a rota basis. There are no domestic staff, as residents and staff are jointly responsible for cleaning, cooking, and routine house maintenance. Weekly community meetings and daily groups are forums for issues concerning the goverment and governance of the houses.

The Fellowship's staff training college not only provides in-service training for Fellowship staff but also provides courses for other interested bodies such as local authority social services departments. Through these and other means, the Fellowship has provided a stimulus to other bodies responsible for halfway houses to develop them along therapeutic community lines. However, such developments have proceeded further in Britain than elsewhere, partly because of bureaucratic requirements elsewhere that such institutions should have a psychiatrist in charge. This is the case in the Netherlands, and although not a requirement in America, the fact that no medical insurance cover is available in care institutions without a physician in charge means that residents may find the cost of a stay in such halfway houses greater than the (reimbursed) cost of a stay in a psychiatric hospital (Hoffman, 1980).

So far we have concentrated our attention on the Richmond Fellowship halfway houses and the local authority houses that the Fellowship has influenced, but the Fellowship is by no means the only organisation in the voluntary sector providing halfway house accommodation following a therapeutic community approach: for example, a number of halfway house communities have been set up catering for alcoholics (for example, Orford et al., 1974). The Simon, Cyrenian, and St Mungo communities caring for vagrants are for the most part approximate to the Rudolf Steiner communities discussed earlier, insofar as the aim is not so much cure or rehabilitation but rather the provision of a caring environment where former denizens of skid row can live with dignity and a sense of worth. However, some of the Cyrenian organisations have also set up halfway houses for former vagrants, prisoners, and common lodging house inmates who wish to return to a 'normal' life.

Laing-ian communities

It would be wrong to end this brief history without some mention of the Laing-ian therapeutic communities, even though these communities are of limited numerical importance. Anyone who can recall the radical sixties, when every bookshelf seemed to hold Laing's *Politics of Experience* (1967) or *The Divided Self* (1960), or who squeezed into crammed halls at 'alternative' venues to hear Laing's dazzling extemporare talks, anyone who can recall that tide of enthusiasm, can only be amazed that its institutional fruits were so small.

Laing and his associates had been working at 'Villa 21' at Shenley Hospital, abandoning Jones-type methods of formal community meetings, a programme of activities, and so on, in favour of a more libertarian approach to the treatment of schizophrenia, which was seen to have a social causation in family relationships (Laing et al.,

1965). However, Cooper, one of Laing's collaborators, has described the difficulties staff faced in attempting to employ such a libertarian approach within the context of a psychiatric hospital; seemingly both administrative and medical colleagues complained repeatedly about the dishevelled state of the buildings in which the community was housed, and the apparent lack of any control of residents by staff. Gradually staff were required to exercise greater authority over residents and Cooper for one felt that it was not possible to develop such techniques to their logical conclusion within the confines of a psychiatric hospital.

In 1965 Laing and his associates managed to lease Kingsley Hall, a Victorian settlement house in London's East End, to provide an environment where schizophrenic patients could heal themselves by psychosis and regression into infancy prior to emotional reconstruction; patients who travelled this journey of 'creative disintegration' could then help other patients to 'heal themselves by becoming sick'. Kingsley Hall's most famous patient was Mary Barnes (Barnes and Berke, 1973). The lease on Kingsley Hall expired in 1970 and the community dispersed: it had been much visited and much written about, but little imitated. The Philadelphia Association (the umbrella organisation which had leased Kingsley Hall) runs a number of Archway communities in short-lease local authority accommodation. Another group from Kingsley Hall (including Joseph Berke, Mary Barnes's 'therapist') set up the Arbours Association (Berke, 1980). Laing himself no longer has a day-to-day involvement in any of these Laing-ian communities.

Institutional psychiatry has long been critical of the Laing-ian approach and this critical comment has continued: for example, Wing (1978) diagnosed Mary Barnes as hysterical rather than schizophrenic. Additional criticism has now come from other therapeutic community practitioners (e.g. Jansen, 1980b) and from the radical left, notably in Sedgwick's book *Psycho Politics* (Sedgwick, 1982). Any further expansion of the Laing-ian communities seems unlikely. Thus the Arbours Association reported the same number of communities (four houses catering for approximately 25 people) in 1985 as Berke had enumerated in 1979.

Conclusion

We will conclude this historical outline with a brief look at the contemporary position of therapeutic communities. In many respects the current situation is an anomalous one. Although a variety of national governments now seem to favour a policy of community care, few seem interested in providing the funding necessary to enable the development of adequate facilities in the community. Certainly it is scandalous that most national governments have refused to provide adequate funding for their ex-psychiatric hospital patients whom the same governments have, for largely financial reasons (Scull, 1977), required the hospitals to discharge. This lack of funding is likely to continue to inhibit the growth of therapeutic communities in the state sector, particularly in day care centres. In those countries (particularly Italy, but also Spain to a lesser extent) where there is an effective political movement, such as the Psichiatrica Democratica, to press for both the closure of the custodial mental hospitals *and* support for community care, there may be a continuing growth of therapeutic communities – but only of certain types. Basaglia, for example, the individual whose name is most closely associated with the Psichiatrica Democratica movement, worked with Maxwell Jones but was rather critical of the Jones-type communities in hospitals, believing, perhaps rather unfairly, that these were an attempt 'to make the asylum work better', whereas his own goal was one of 'laying the groundwork for its total destruction' (Basaglia, 1981). However, the Psichiatrica Democratica movement arose in Italy out of a distinctive alliance between left-wing politics and psychiatry, and as Sedgwick (1982) has pointed out, it is inconceivable that anything approximating to that movement could occur in Britain or America. Indeed, as Dalley (1983) has recently argued, community care, within the British context at least, has had rather more to do with assuming the family to be the proper locus of care than with creating alternative radical structures within the community.

Nevertheless, the very inadequacy of state and local government programmes of care *may* help to nurture voluntary bodies like the Camphill movement and the Richmond Fellowship: where existing state and municipal facilities are inadequate, central and local government will perhaps be more willing to fund places in the voluntary sector which are able, as a result of their independent status, to experiment with therapeutic community methods. However, only some types of communities would benefit from this: residential psychiatric units organised as therapeutic communities, despite their intellectual vigour, are likely to continue to face difficulties, and various forms of residential community treatment like the concept houses, which compete with alternative (and cheaper) day care provision, may also come to face funding problems. Geel-type communities for the boarding of the disabled and the disturbed will probably continue to gain ground in southern Europe, where they are advocated by the Psichiatrica Democratica movement. If they are to become more common in Britain similar advocacy is required: it is perhaps an encouraging start that authorities as diverse as John Wing (from academic psychiatry) and Peter Sedgwick (from the Marxist left) have set their seal of approval on Geel.

Chapter 2
The settings

Introduction

In this chapter we shall try to provide some information on the communities included in our comparative study. However, rather than list the bare facts of each setting (size, location, funding, and so on – which would be exceedingly tedious), we shall try instead to convey something of what life was like within each community.

Such descriptions can only be subjective impressions. We have chosen to base our descriptions on our own experiences as incoming researchers, simply in order for the reader to glimpse something of what it was like for a newcomer to live and work within each of these settings.

The Camphill Rudolf Steiner Community

Camphill was by far the largest, and in some respects the most unusual, setting included in our study (McKeganey, 1982). The community was formed in 1939 when a small group of Austrian refugees, fleeing Nazi persecution, arrived in the north east of Scotland to apply the religious and philosophical principles of the Austrian mystic, philosopher, and teacher Rudolf Steiner (1861–1925) in the formation of a residential community for handicapped children. As most readers will be unfamiliar with Steiner's ideas, we will devote rather more attention here to the Camphill community than to our other settings.

Today, Camphill exists as a number of individual house communities dotted around three model village estates in the countryside surrounding a Scottish city. Walking around these estates one has a clear sense of the European origins of the community – where grey, granite stone prevails in the nearby city, within the community there is a preponderance of natural woods and Swiss-style, white-painted house fronts. Furthermore, many of the buildings show evidence of Steiner's ideas on architecture, with the central hall, for example, resembling a large dome-like plant. Physically, then, Camphill looks very distinctive.

Initial images of rural tranquillity, however, are likely to be quickly dispelled by the appearance of many children, whose animated welcome involves a seemingly unending list of questions: Is that your car? Does it have a radio? Does it work? And the inevitable – can I listen to it?

As a newcomer one may only gradually become aware of the individual handicaps of the various children: the socially inept and inarticulate child hanging on the sidelines, or the initially animated, aphasic child, who greets one with a smile and an embrace only to run away when questioned lest his handicap be revealed. At first sight Camphill may appear to be a village made up entirely of children; in fact, there were over one hundred and sixty adult co-workers living and working with the children.

There were several distinctive anthroposophical therapies provided for the children, which were very much a part of Camphill. McKeganey, for example, well remembers the acute sense of culture shock he experienced when his arrival coincided with one of the children's music and coloured light therapy sessions. He recorded the events in his fieldnotes for the day:

> I arrived today and following brief introductions to some of the co-workers was shown immediately into a darkened room in which a number of adults were sat facing a translucent drape hanging at one end. I noticed that each of the walls, including the door through which I had entered, were all covered by long curtains, giving the room a curious, cocoon-like appearance. After some moments a child was shown into the room and sat in a single chair in front of the adults and facing the translucent drape. An adult in one corner began to play on a harp-like musical instrument and the room was filled with a diffused purple light. From behind the screen an adult began a series of ballet-like movements and as she did so the purple light was successively changed to red, yellow, blue, etc. When finally the room lights were switched on it was explained that the child had

> been experiencing considerable difficulty incarnating into her body, and that the music and coloured lights were an attempt to create a sense of the spirit world in the room – the idea being that this might encourage the child to strengthen her attachment to the physical world.

Welcome as it was, this explanation only heightened McKeganey's sense of incomprehension about what had happened in the room. Indeed, to have understood what had taken place it would have been necessary to have known something of Rudolf Steiner's anthroposophical ideas on health, illness and therapy, since it was these ideas which informed much of what happened within the community (McKeganey, 1983).

According to Steiner, human development has principally to do with a process of incarnating from the spirit world to the physical world. Each of us has, it is maintained, a spiritual body which is in constant activity within one's physical body, fashioning it and developing it in accordance with one's spiritual destiny. The physical body itself, according to Steiner, is little more than the shell upon which our spirit forces operate:

> The body which we have from birth till the change of first teeth is, in a sense, nothing else than a model we take over from our parents: it contains the forces of heredity, our forefathers have helped to build it. In the course of the first seven years we thrust off this body. A completely new body comes into being: the body that man has after the change of teeth is not built up by the forces of heredity but entirely by the spirit-and-soul which has descended. (Steiner, 1972, p. 25)

Although the physical changes a child undergoes in the first few years of life are among the most obvious signs of this incarnating process, in fact, according to Steiner, incarnating activity takes place throughout the entire course of one's life. So, for example, when one falls asleep at night, a part of one's spirit centre leaves the physical body and temporarily returns to the spirit world.

Although in the case of normal children one is largely unaware of this incarnating activity taking place, this does not apply with handicapped children, since, for one reason or another, their spirit forces have been unable to enter into their physical body correctly. Steiner describes a number of conditions which, he says, are the manifestations of difficulties occurring in the child's incarnation from the spirit world; the epileptic child, for example, is cited as one in which the spirit forces have become 'jammed up' in the human body, while, conversely, the hysterical child is seen as one whose spirit forces are passing too easily through his or her body. In fact, Steiner describes a wide range of developmental handicaps in children which, he says, are the direct result of difficulties occurring in the incarnating process, for example, nocturnal enuresis: 'Whenever you have a case of bed-wetting, you can assume that the astral body is running out, is overflowing.' (Steiner, 1972, p. 78)

Seen in those terms, childhood handicaps are regarded pre-eminently as a spiritual phenomenon. Even the most profoundly handicapped of children is seen as having an inviolate spiritual centre which is struggling to enter into, and come to terms with, a weakened physical body. It is perhaps this single idea, more than any other, which is at the root of so much of the community's work – discovering that centre in each child and facilitating its incarnation into the child's physical body.

While these ideas are apparent in the many distinctive anthroposophical therapies provided for the children, like, for example, the coloured light treatment, they are also very influential in many other aspects of life within the community. A good deal of emphasis is placed upon establishing warm and close ties between the children and the adult co-workers in the belief that this is one way of encouraging the spiritual centre within each child to develop to its fullest potential. A former medical superintendent at Camphill has provided a secular description of the importance of these ideas in discussing the relationships between adults and handicapped children:

> We might see the handicapped child as an artist who has to play on a faulty instrument. Even when we ask the finest of pianists to play on an unsound instrument ... his performance will be a bad one. Those in the audience who have had little musical experience will think that he is a bad artist. Displeasure and disappointment will show on their faces and the artist will be unable to give of his best ... on the other hand, if some in the audience are musically sensitive and know the piece ... they will perceive his intentions and interpretation ... his performance will improve and the concert may turn out to be a considerable success. (Weihs, 1971, p. 35)

In order to develop close ties the adults both live and work alongside the children. Dormitory parents, for example, will often have their own room adjacent to the children's dormitory. They will wake the children each morning, dress them, have breakfast with them, take them to and from the community school, look after them in the evenings, take them out on trips or outings over the weekend, and on Sunday accompany them to the central hall for a religious ceremony. The dormitory parents can quite literally be with the children for twenty-four hours a day.

Needless to say, such close contact can be exhausting for the adults and it is not surprising that many of the dormitory parents only remain in the community for between one and two years. The relative impermanence of dormitory parents is itself seen as being of therapeutic value:

> A very favourable factor at work in temporary or impermanent group mothers and fathers is that possessive relationships are not so easily built up between adult and child. A free, warm reciprocal relationship between group and group parent is the most beneficial. (Weihs, 1971, p. 160)

The emphasis within each of the house communities is on maintaining as normal a domestic environment as possible. In addition to the dormitory parents, there are the more permanent house parents, for whom the house is quite literally their home. Throughout the community there are no salaried staff, no shifts, no sense of a Monday-to-Friday working week, and all finances are organised on a single household basis. All of this is very much in accordance with Steiner's ideas on community living:

> In a community of human beings working together the well-being of the community will be the greater the less the individual claims for himself the proceeds of the work he has himself done, i.e. the more of these proceeds he makes over to his fellow workers, and the more his own requirements are satisfied, not out of his own work done, but out of the work done by others. (Steiner, 1958, p. 32)

In addition to the important part played by such warm ties between the adults and children, considerable emphasis is also placed on the potential for developing therapeutic relationships between the children. It is frequently noted, for example, that children with quite different handicaps can often offer each other help more spontaneously than can adults. For this reason an attempt is made to combine a therapeutic range of handicaps in each house and dormitory. Again the former medical superintendent:

> The community has generally learned to recognise and, I would say, give the fullest possible play to the unique help that one child can give another. That which the mongol can give to the autistic and vice-versa, or the mutual assistance afforded between the maladjusted and the physically disabled. This help is often more spontaneous and instinctive than adults are inclined to think, and when it is given the opportunity to unfold it becomes a creative therapeutic force within the whole. (Weihs, 1971, p. 159)

Although it is relatively easy to show the sense of bewilderment a new arrival may feel in the community, it is also the case that many of the routines and activities that seemed odd or strange at first very quickly became an accepted and even welcomed part of one's day. In conversation with community members during his first day, for example, the importance of maintaining a rhythmic ascending-descending structure to each day was explained to McKeganey. Such a structure was seen as essential for assisting the child's incarnation from the spirit world. Hardly giving these ideas much further thought, McKeganey was surprised the following morning when he was woken at 6.30 a.m. by one of the adults playing a recorder in the corridor outside his room – this, it was explained, was the beginning of that ascending structure. Similarly, at the end of the evening there was an elaborate 'settling' procedure which represented the conclusion of the descending structure. Typically this involved the dormitory parent going over the various events of the day with the children as they lay in bed. This would be followed by a candle-lit story, a short piece of lyre or guitar music, and finally a prayer.

At first McKeganey regarded these rituals with little more than a vague sense of impatience, eager as he often was to get on and talk to the co-workers about their work in the community. Quite quickly, however, he came to appreciate the structured orderliness of these routines and to suspend his own desire always to be 'doing something else'.

In the early stages of his fieldwork McKeganey also regarded it as rather odd and somewhat irksome that, along with the other adults, he would frequently have to dress the children in their 'Sunday best' and accompany them to a classical music recital held in the main hall. For many of the children it was simply too much for them to sit quietly for an hour or so and listen to the music. Gradually, however, McKeganey began to accept the house-parents' explanation that the music would often touch the children's inner centre even if outwardly they appeared not to be listening. He also came to regard his earlier attitude as being based on little more than prejudice.

It is very difficult to say exactly what influence Steiner's ideas had on the children, most of whom had been referred by local authorities for a wide range of problems. The organisers of the community, however, were very keen to ensure that the children should experience life outside the community and to this end required the children to return to their own homes or to the care of their local authority for the duration of the school holidays. Apart from allowing the adults a much needed rest, these periods were also held to be important in broadening the children's experience of the outside world.

The day hospital community

Set in the grounds of a large psychiatric hospital, the Ross Clinic provided day care for approximately thirty patients diagnosed as neurotic or personality-disordered. Although most of the patients attended the hospital on a day basis there were a few in-patients. Staff in the day hospital consisted of four psychiatrists and one occupational therapist, each of whom had responsibilities outside the unit, and four full-time psychiatric nurses and a regular throughput of final year medical students (Bloor, 1980, 1981; McKeganey and Bloor, 1987; Morrice, 1973).

In common with some of the other settings included in our study, referrals to the community had dropped off; at one point in the fieldwork, for example, patient numbers were as low as eight. Most of the patients arrived at the day hospital following some kind of personal or social crisis, for example, attempted suicide or marital breakdown. While it was an agreed part of the admission policy that patients would only be accepted following the establishment of a 'contract' as to the nature of their problems and their preparedeness to 'work' on these in the groups, in fact relatively few referrals were ever turned down.

To an outsider – new patient, visitor or researcher – arrival at the day hospital was an unsettling experience. New patients would be handed a printed sheet detailing the programme and told little more than that all treatment took place in the groups, of which there were a bewildering number: a community meeting each morning, twice-weekly activity groups for such things as gardening and cooking, twice-weekly occupational therapy sessions, daily small groups, and a weekly encounter group. In addition there were a variety of daily and weekly staff groups.

It was not simply the number of groups that was bewildering for the new arrival. There was also something rather unsettling in the *way* patients spoke to each other both within and outside of the groups. Although people were certainly very friendly, their conversations often rang strange: intimate disclosures, uncomfortable silences and weeping denunciations were familiar occurrences. Similarly, people often seemed to spend as much time concentrating upon why a person had said something as on what it was they had said. It was not easy to predict responses: a tearful confession might be described as attention-seeking at just the point that one had thought of offering a word of sympathy or a comforting hand.

Appeals for guidance or advice, while not falling on deaf ears, were hardly helped by suggestions like 'just say what feels right'. Bloor still recalls the mortification he felt during the pilot study when he apologised to one of the nurses for his silence in the group by explaining that he had been uncertain as to what to say for the best. The nurse gave him a kindly smile and said 'Poor Mick: he wanted to be therapeutic so he said nothing, eh?'

This initial sense of strangeness should not be over-emphasised since new arrivals were often able to function at a minimum level by 'going through the motions' even if they did not entirely understand the nature of what it was they were doing. One newly arrived patient, for example, conducted himself with apparent competence in the encounter group, only to mutter to Bloor afterwards 'What the hell's going on?' Overcoming this sense of strangeness was, as we shall see in Chapter Three, a central part of the treatment process. It was often possible to hear senior patients and staff reminiscing (perhaps for the benefit of a new arrival) about their own initial terror, now lost, of speaking in the groups and showing their own feelings.

The average length of stay of patients who did not default from treatment was about three and a half months.

Parkneuk

Parkneuk was the first community studied by Bloor and the one with which our comparative study began. It is difficult to say precisely why Parkneuk was such an attractive place to visit. Partly it had to do with the rather idyllic setting of the community in a large family house in the Scottish countryside, partly, though, it had to do with the foster family approach to therapy adopted within the community. Entering Parkneuk was rather like entering a large family home.

Although as a new arrival one was well aware of a formal order of routines these tended to be of a domestic rather than an obviously 'therapeutic' nature; there were no formal group therapy meetings and only occasional planned activities. Instead, the boarders' day was very much taken up with such things as looking after the house, preparing the meals, working in the field, or spending time in the weavery.

While visitors were made very welcome, there was a recognition that their arrival must not become a disruption. So, for example, a boarder keen to show the visitor the new piglets would be reminded to finish setting the table first. In the meantime one of the adult co-workers would most likely introduce the visitor to another resident too shy to initiate conversation him or herself. Therapeutic considerations tended to be interwoven with the domestic routines of the house. Notice the managed sociability found in the following fieldnote:

> When I went over to borrow the trolley-jack, Robert (co-worker) and I spent a long time on the front steps chewing the fat about this and that. Vera, Len, Victor and Ken all came and went as well as friends and neighbours. Throughout this the talk broadened and narrowed in a natural manner: with Ken (Down's Syndrome boy) there was some buffoonery around the issues of dressing him in his coat and wellies and offering him some of Kim and Larry's sweets; with Victor (withdrawn schizophrenic) there was an exchange of polite conversational pleasantries. These social events occurred naturally but, simultaneously, the boarders were consciously attended to – they were consciously drawn into natural social events.

In certain respects Parkneuk resembled the Camphill community described above, and while some of the current co-workers disclaimed any knowledge of Steiner's ideas, all of the original co-workers had, at one time or another, worked within Steiner communities. As at Camphill, a good deal of emphasis was placed on the benefits of co-workers and boarders actually living together. There were no salaries, and no shifts, though (as at Camphill) co-workers were allocated one free day each week. So thorough-going was this sense of communalism that Bloor recalled how difficult it was for many of the adults to create the backstage privacy to answer his questions about the boarders.

This communalism, however, should not be confused with a formal democracy, since only relatively few, if any, of the residents showed any interest in the management of the community. Similarly, although there was a general agreement that formal meetings of co-workers ought to be held, in fact such meetings were the exception rather than the rule, and decision-making tended to be emergent, consensual, and involved mutual accommodation.

As at Camphill, a good deal of importance was placed on maintaining a range of handicaps in the house so as to allow the boarders maximum scope in helping each other. Similarly, as at Camphill, much was made of the therapeutic benefits of a routine ordering of activities in the house. Bloor, for example, noted the importance of what he described at the time as 'benign routines' (Bloor, 1980):

> Lunchtime has a smooth, routine quality. After the meal there is a holding of hands and intoning of 'Thank you for the meal'. Everybody rises unbidden and carries the crockery and such-like through to the kitchen. The scraps are recovered for the dog or pig. Someone (one of the co-workers) starts to wash up and those boarders on the rota pick up the tea towels and begin to wipe up. Even Ken (Down's Syndrome boy) usually starts wiping up unbidden, taking up his favourite place by the stove. Someone else makes coffee. There is no regimentation – events have a naturalistic family-like occurrence. Afterwards people quickly melt off to their rooms for a short break before work starts again at 2.30.

Boarders at Parkneuk were actively encouraged to mix socially with the community's neighbours and could frequently be seen attending functions in the local village hall, or visiting the home of the local postmistress to watch *Top of the Pops* on her television.

The activity basis of therapeutic work within Parkneuk derived from the fact that many of the boarders were recruited at age sixteen from Camphill with the intention of equipping them with the necessary domestic and working skills to enable them to graduate to an adult anthroposophical community (like Newton Dee), where they would be required to take their place as useful members of the community.

Just as the boarders could develop particular skills and interests in the course of their residence at Parkneuk, so also could the co-workers. The pursuit of these interests could be a source of considerable 'job satisfaction' to co-workers, who did not in the main have a sacrificial or altruistic approach to their boarders, but rather were willing to share their lives with the disturbed and handicapped in return for the perceived rewards of a communal lifestyle and for the opportunity to pursue and develop absorbing interests. The co-workers had a trade-off motivation, kindred to that of the Flemish townspeople in Geel. Some co-workers, when they left Parkneuk, sold their new-won skills in the market-place; thus the herb-grower eventually left with his wife, child, and one of the boarders, to run his own herb garden and dried flower business.

Faswells

Like the Ross Clinic, Faswells was located within the grounds of a large psychiatric hospital. However, unlike at the Ross Clinic, its host institution was depressingly traditional. Set on the outskirts of London, its high perimeter wall and huge gates were a dull reminder of its custodial past. The community itself was situated in a rather shabby bungalow erected at the furthest corner of the hospital grounds. Physically, the building was little more than a long corridor, at various points along which were the small group rooms, kitchen, office, and such-like, leading to the large lounge and two large dormitories.

At the time of the study there were fifteen members resident within the unit (with space for a further five), most of whom were diagnosed as neurotic or personality-disordered. According to the Faswells consultant there had been a general drop-off in referrals to the community, with the consequence that some residents had been accepted for treatment even though their suitability for therapeutic community-type work could be questioned.

Staffing at Faswells was similar to that at the Ross, with four psychiatrists, all of whom had commitments outside the community, and seven full-time psychiatric nurses. The formal programme was a mixture of large and small group meetings, weekly art and music therapy sessions, and a 'work and leaving' group.

Whereas at the Ross there was a sense of things happening, within Faswells it was more one of things having happened in the rather distant past. This was apparent early on in McKeganey's fieldwork when he attended a staff meeting at which many of the staff expressed disquiet at the apparent lack of any sense of direction or progress within the community. It was noted, for example, that the average length of stay among the current resident group was two years, that this was far too long, and indicative of a lack of understanding as to what was expected of residents. It was also suggested that modifying the formal programme and introducing such things as a communal meal, a psycho-drama group, and a dream therapy session, would go some way towards injecting new life into the community. Accompanying this, however, was a feeling that each of these ideas had been suggested at times in the past without ever having come to fruition.

As a new arrival one very quickly picked up a sense of uninterest amongst many of the residents. With the conclusion of the formal programme in the evenings and at weekends it seemed that residents could not wait to leave the unit. McKeganey noted with some dismay his own experience of remaining in the community over a weekend period:

> I decided to remain in the unit this weekend to see what it was like. For much of today (Saturday) the place has been empty. Various of the residents have drifted in for meals and at odd times throughout the day. For the most part though I've sat watching TV or chatting to the nurses – all of whom have sympathised with me on the prospect of staying through till Monday morning!

Although residents were expected to clean certain areas of the unit, for much of the time the building remained in a pretty dishevelled state, and most of the work fell to a hospital-appointed cleaner. In addition, residents showed a general reluctance to participate in any kind of therapeutic discussion outside the small groups and selected large groups. Following a particularly quiet large group meeting, for example, one of the nurses commented bitterly: 'I don't see how I can justify my work here when all [the residents] do is clockwatch. When the psychiatrists are not there you have to spoon-feed the discussion to them all the time and even then they do nothing.' Equally, there were many occasions when residents would comment, in the company of nurses, that they could see little point in discussing sensitive or potentially threatening material unless the psychiatrists were present.

The impression given at Faswells, then, was less that of a group therapy setting, more one of private communication between residents and individual psychiatrists. It should be pointed out here that while staff at Faswells broadly accepted McKeganey's description of their community, nevertheless it was felt that the study had coincided with a period when the community was at a particularly low point and was, in some senses at least, rather atypical of itself (McKeganey, 1984b, 1986; McKeganey and Bloor, 1987).

Ravenscroft

Like the Faswells community, Ravenscroft was located within the grounds of a fairly traditional psychiatric hospital set on the outskirts of London. The unit provided short-to-medium stay residential care on a five-day-week basis to a client group diagnosed as neurotic or personality-disordered. Frankly psychotic patients were not accepted for treatment.

At the time of the study there were twelve residents within the unit, though there was space for a further three. The average age of this group was thirty-four. The expected length of residence at the time of the study was six months.

Staffing at Ravenscroft was similar to that at Ross and Faswells: there were two psychiatrists, a senior psychologist, an art therapist, a social worker, and various nurses, all of whom, apart from the nurses, had additional commitments outside the unit. Once again the formal programme consisted of a combination of large and small group meetings, art therapy sessions, periodic resident reviews, and some planned and unplanned social activities.

While in terms of structure, hospital location, and client group, Ravenscroft resembled Faswells, in all other respects the two settings were very different (McKeganey, 1984b, 1986). Though set in the hospital grounds, the community itself was located in what at one time had been the home of the medical superintendent. Far from resembling a psychiatric ward, Ravenscroft looked more like a large family home. Similarly, whereas Faswells had two large dormitories, Ravenscroft residents shared a room with only one or two others. The internal decor and furnishings had an obviously 'homely' appearance which further reduced the clinical appearance of the unit.

As was the case at Parkneuk, many of the routines within Ravenscroft were domestic rather than overtly therapeutic. Cleaning and some minor household repairs, for example, were the residents' responsibilities, as was purchasing and preparing food for meals. However, whereas the emphasis at Parkneuk was on accomplishing activities that were regarded as therapeutic in themselves, for example, cooking or working in the field, at Ravenscroft such domestic activities were seen as providing a mass of material for subsequent discussion in the formal groups. Early on in the fieldwork McKeganey attended one large group discussion that was almost entirely devoted to deciding upon the membership of the various cooking groups. Suddenly, and without any apparent warning, one of the residents began hurling abuse at a fellow member, who, it was alleged, was not doing his share of the work. Staff and fellow residents, however, channelled the individual's anger into a consideration of what he wanted from other people. Staff also invited him to consider whether the anger he felt towards the other resident was in fact a reflection of the unresolved anger he felt towards his father.

In part, it was this potential for weaving therapeutic discussions out of apparently mundane activities that could be the most unsettling feature of life at Ravenscroft. As was also true for the Ross Clinic, such discussions often extended beyond the formal groups. There were numerous occasions when residents would continue discussing material raised in the formal groups, either in the evening, sitting around the kitchen table, or in the nearby public house. These discussions would often be fed back into the formal groups the following day by the residents themselves or by whichever of the regular Ravenscroft nurses had been taking his or her turn on the overnight rota.

Whereas at Faswells one had a sense of therapy being a feature of one-to-one interchanges between individual residents and individual members of staff, at Ravenscroft the impression was rather more of a dynamic and internally cohesive community where residents spent a good deal of time discussing and responding to one another's difficulties.

Ashley House

This community was located in a large old house close to the centre of a provincial English town. Like Ravenscroft and Parkneuk, Ashley looked more like a large family home than a therapeutic community. Residents and staff had responsibility for both the domestic routines within the house and the internal decorations.

The house had space for fourteen residents, most of whom stayed for around four months. Referrals came mainly from the social work and probation services, many of the residents having experienced difficulties coping with adverse family circumstances or with adjustment following stays in custodial or psychiatric institutions. Staff there consisted of a warden, a deputy and three other adult workers including a 'trainee scholar' (trainee staff who received in-service training on a day-release basis for a two-year period). From time to time there were also social work students attending the house on a placement basis. Staff within Ashley operated a rota whereby they would take their turn sleeping overnight within the unit.

Although in certain respects the house resembled a large family home, in certain other respects the atmosphere was quite distinctive. For example, the adolescent residents showed a relaxed, open solicitude towards visitors, but they were often openly abusive or aggressive to one another. While such behaviour is probably common within adolescent peer groups it is not often openly displayed in the company of adults. On some occasions these exchanges would amount to little more than good-humoured banter and sexual innuendo, but on others they could take on a more aggressive or even menacing character.

Staff generally eschewed any kind of authoritarian clamping down on such behaviour, preferring instead to encourage residents themselves to exercise individual and collective restraint. Nevertheless, Bloor recorded his own sense of being at a loss to know how to react to residents' outbursts, and in the early stages of his fieldwork frequently found himself feigning the need to attend to important domestic business elsewhere in the house. Only gradually did he learn to cope with these outbursts in the way that the staff did, by deprecating them not from a position of authority, but of a fellow community member whose domestic peace was being violated.

It was staff practice to work largely in reaction to events in the community, rather than indulge in any detailed planning of therapeutic interventions. As a consequence, staff were often unable to set aside time for socialising with visitors or new staff, and were often unable to provide anything other than the most general statements as to how one should conduct oneself in the groups ('just say what feels right'). New arrivals, though, were likely to remain fearful of behaving in an unplanned or unscripted way, and were understandably uncertain of what their feelings were.

The house programme at Ashley consisted of a weekly community meeting, daily work groups for cleaning the house, and coffee groups during which the residents' activities in the previous work groups would be discussed. On most afternoons residents involved themselves in individual or group projects, for example, laying out a war-game in the basement, though they could, if they wished, attend the staff feedback meeting or the first part of the weekly staff meeting (dealing with administrative issues). In addition to their participation in these meetings some of the residents were involved in activities outside the house – employment (part- or full-time), voluntary work, or part- or full-time education.

Residents seemed to enjoy the democratic ethos of the house and often contrasted it favourably with more authoritarian institutions with which they had previously been familiar. As a result of the residents' willingness to participate in the groups staff were able to renounce a supervisory role. Staff ensured the adequate running of the community by indirect means, by encouraging individual and collective resident responsibilities – staff 'orchestrated' the running of the house.

Beeches House

Beeches House was in some ways very similar to Ashley, and in others quite different. Run by the same charitable trust, the house provided residential care for a similar, though not identical, client group – a greater proportion of the adolescent residents at Beeches were classifiable as educationally subnormal. Like Ashley, Beeches was located in a large house, though in the suburbs, rather than the centre, of a large provincial town. The staffing was similar in both houses, though at Beeches there was a qualified teacher.

The feature of Beeches which distinguished it from Ashley and also from all of the other communities included in our study, was in the degree of planning of activities. Where visitors to Ashley often found themselves being swept along with the onrush of events, at Beeches there was rather more of a sense of being inducted into an efficient, well-oiled, smooth-running system. New arrivals were allocated a fellow resident (the buddy system), whose job it was to show them round the house, explain the programme, and generally look after them at meal times. House activities were carefully planned in advance and executed in the way of a well-ordered routine.

The level of planning was a fundamental principle of therapy. Some understanding of the extent and pervasiveness of this planning can be seen in the following extract from the staff's 'operations manual', which described the 45-minute staff pre-meeting that preceded the weekly community meeting:

> The final 30 minutes is to be spent reviewing the dynamics of the community. It is important here that the staff team can decide on any necessary consequences for any specific resident behaviour and, where possible, reach agreement on a consistent staff attitude and intervention. If a matter is to be raised by staff it should decided by whom and how it is to be raised. If any particular resident is going to be put 'on the hot seat' through heavy criticism for unacceptable behaviour, care must be taken that that resident is not left feeling completely demoralised. To avoid this it is necessary to make sure that something positive is said about that resident. (This must not be fabricated but something genuinely worthwhile that person has done.)

Note that beyond legislating for consistent staff interventions, the manual also anticipated residents' reactions (demoralisation), outlined a remedy (praise for something positive), and guarded against abuse (no fabrication). Significantly, it was not simply the formal programme that was planned in this way but also the residents' leisure time and even holiday activities.

The house programme consisted of work groups every morning bar Sunday, followed by morning meetings for the discussion of residents' conduct in the group, allocating residents' tasks around the house, and reviewing any problems or issues that had surfaced since the previous day. In addition, there were compulsory weekly community meetings, an all-resident meeting for discussion of a single (rotating) resident, and a staff pre-meeting preceding the community meeting. As at Ashley, a number of the Beeches residents were also involved in full- or part-time work outside the community.

Although newcomers might find the extensiveness of the house structure initially confusing and taxing on the memory they soon developed a practised grasp of the house and their place within it. Bloor recalled in an early fieldnote his well-meant attempts to prod a resident, with whom he had cleaned the dining room, into disclosing to the morning meeting the information that he and Bloor had located a pile of rotting cornflakes behind the dresser. The resident, however, shushed Bloor with the correction that the meeting was only in its first stage, the resident chairman's report, and the matter of the rotting cornflakes ought to be raised at a later point.

In addition to the general planning of activities within the house, there was also a carefully devised structure of formal statuses, with attendant duties and privileges, through which residents progressed. Since residents were expected to work their way up through this formal status hierarchy, staff generally expected them to stay in the house for between one and two years. In reality, however, this expectation was rarely met, since most of the residents left prematurely either as a result of failing to settle in the house, or because of funding difficulties, or because of offences requiring custodial treatment. Fuller accounts of both Ashley and Beeches can be found in Bloor, 1984, 1986a, and 1986b.

The concept house

The community was housed in a large building in a Dutch city. The neighbourhood was an affluent one but it abutted a run-down, inner-city area; several neighbouring houses had been turned to institutional uses.

When Fonkert arrived at the house to begin his research he was feeling anxious and ill; subsequent events did not improve his state of mind. He was immediately placed on 'the stool', an uncomfortable, wooden, child's chair in the front hallway. He sat there for over an hour, forbidden to speak with anyone, smiling and nodding at the preoccupied occupants of the house scurrying past him, bellowing out to each other, as they went about their business. He then entered the 'intake' phase of the house programme: he went into an office where five people fired questions at him more rapidly than he could possibly answer, he exchanged his clothes for house overalls, he submitted to a haircut, and finally he was asked to demonstrate a commitment to the house – somebody (knowing he was newly married) suggested he surrender his wedding ring. He had entered therapy.

New residents were kept completely incommunicado (no letters, no phone calls, no private conversations). There was a complex and strenuous weekly programme designed to keep residents busy and under pressure encountering situations designed to exceed their ability to cope. There were different departments: kitchen, housekeeping, gardening/construction, administration/public relations, a separate department for new arrivals, and, at the base of the social pyramid, 'the washing tub' for those who were 'acting out'. Each department had its own hierarchy of crew-members, assistant foreman, and foreman. Above the departmental foremen were the expeditors (house police), the head expeditor, and the coordinator. All these positions (including overnight supervision – 'the nightwatch') were shared out amongst the thirty to forty residents. Staff, of whom there were eight (including a social worker and a full-time administrator, and excluding a psychiatrist available on a consultative basis), were not part of this structure – the residents themselves maintained and policed the concept house, monitored by the staff. (For a comprehensive description of the programme and structure, see Fonkert, 1978; for a description of a comparable British concept house, see Kennard, 1976.)

The concept house was a pressure cooker: high standards of work were required, supervision was strict, criticisms ('pull-ups', 'haircuts', and denunciations in the encounter groups) were commonplace and directed as frequently towards attitudes as towards behaviour. The rules were highly restrictive: for example, all socialising had to be conducted in groups rather than pairs, and, additionally, staff had recourse to 'therapeutic measures' such as requiring residents to carry a signboard proclaiming their transgressions ('I have brought the values of the street into the community'), as well as demotion in the hierarchy and loss of privileges. The aim was to precipitate catharsis and strip the addict of a favourable self-image. In return, the resident was offered warm, affectionate and 'honest' relationships and praise for his or her achievements (the 'positive' haircut).

The mechanism for behavioural change was for addicts to act 'as if', to conduct themselves in all their activities and relationships *as if* they were the reconstructed being whom the house desired to turn out, to act repeatedly *as if* they were that being until new attitudes and patterns of behaviour became ingrained by repetition and unthinkingly adopted for their own.

Some concept houses also pursued specialist therapies. Fonkert's study community engaged in bio-energetics, in meditations (beginning at five in the morning!) based on the teachings of Bagwan Shri Rajneesh, and in 'scream groups' based on Janov's work on the 'primal scream' (Janov, 1973).

The concept house was itself part of a wider network of local care institutions for the addict population; the house's referrals and discharges were channelled through this wider network. Most referrals came to the house from a local intake/detoxification unit, where a decision would be taken on whether the person would derive most benefit from residential treatment (the concept house) or from a day centre (see Bremer et al., 1977). Discharge normally occurred between one and two years after referral; discharged residents went to a halfway house, normally for a period of a year, and often worked in the concept house as a volunteer staff-member. On 're-entry' (departure from the halfway house) many residents took up paid staff posts in concept houses. Other components of this local network of treatment facilities were street-based social workers and a walk-in counselling service.

The concept house was supported by grants from the Ministry of Health and the Ministry of Social Welfare. Residents also contributed fees from their welfare benefits, collected at source by the house social worker.

This concludes our introductory description of the various communities. In the following chapter we shall concentrate on the contrast between Ashley and Beeches in order to elucidate the different approaches to therapy found in different communities.

Chapter 3

Reality construction, reality confrontation and instrumentalism

At the core of the therapeutic community approach is the induction of the incoming resident into a new social world emphatically different from the resident's old world. Residents encounter not just a new physical environment and new social relationships, but new ways of seeing and describing social life and their place in it. They soon realise that a therapeutic community is not 'just another' treatment setting with new faces occupying old statuses and performing old roles, where they can conduct themselves much as in the past and treatment is a technical accomplishment of specialists. In the therapeutic community, modification of the resident's social conduct, and with it his or her ways of relating to others and his or her felt social identity, *is* the treatment.

It is mere bathos to remark that resocialisation of the individual is no easy matter; there is likely to be considerable resistance to the adoption of a new social world which conflicts explicitly or implicitly with the tenets of an old social world imbibed semi-automatically in childhood and possibly reinforced by much subsequent experience. So resocialisation of the individual is both the core of the treatment approach and a problematic aspect of therapeutic community practice. Any agency that undertakes resocialisation with any success (the armed services and religious sects are oft-cited examples) is likely to have developed particular pedagogic techniques to accomplish that goal. Therapeutic communities are no exception to this rule, but different communities have developed quite different resocialisation techniques. Indeed, the techniques used in some communities are almost antithetically opposed to the techniques used in other communities.

In some of our communities resocialisation proceeded largely through the creation of a controlled environment and the close supervision of resident task performance within that environment, so that behavioural change was called forth and reinforced by the social structure of the community. We will call this approach 'instrumentalism' since behavioural change is effected not by direct appeal but indirectly through the instrument of the social structure, and it occurs not by an effort of resident will but by the unnoticed accretion of experience. In other communities, in contrast, socialisation proceeded largely by the repetitive portrayal to residents of their conduct as unacceptable and by appeals for a volitional change of conduct, coupled with the depiction of the community as a locale where other, less pathogenic, ways of behaving could be experimented with and adopted. We will follow other writers on therapeutic communities (notably Morrice, 1979), in calling this approach 'reality confrontation'; although the term has connotations of angry denunciation, in practice the reflection back to individuals of others' views of their behaviour may encompass a broad spectrum of discourse from hesitant concern through gentle irony to righteous anger.

We shall amplify this instrumentalism/reality confrontation distinction by a detailed examination of contrasting practices in two communities, Beeches and Ashley, from which it will be evident that our distinction is one of emphasis rather than of kind, so that we can go on to place each of our study communities in terms of their relative emphasis on, and particular adaptation of, each of these two approaches. But this empirical examination of socialisation techniques will be preceded by an attempt to place the nature and problems of socialisation into the therapeutic community in a more general sociological context.

Reality construction and the therapeutic community

The sociological study of the socialisation process was transformed in the 1960s by the posthumous publication of the collected papers of the philosopher Alfred Schutz (see especially Schutz, 1962; 1964) and of the subsequent widely read book by Peter Berger (one of Schutz's former students) and Thomas Luckmann, *The Social Construction of Reality*. Starting from an interest in the nature and structure of everyday or 'commonsense' knowledge, Schutz emphasised the massively conservative character of subjective reality – its resistance to radical transformation.

The various aspects of residents' everyday knowledge of the social world which make for resistance to resocialisation can be briefly sketched. First, the residents' everyday social world is a shared one: very little of our everyday knowledge originates in our own experience; most of it is taken over lock, stock and barrel – interpretations, vocabularies, and affective colourations – from others. And these others – family, friends, and workmates – validate and reinforce the reality of that social world for the resident.

Secondly, the residents' subjective reality is no perilous perch, continually wobbling under repeated scrutiny and existential doubt, but is largely taken for granted and is only occasionally and unusually open for reinspection in the light of alternative and competing interpretations. As a consequence of this taken-for-granted quality, the residents' everyday knowledge contains all sorts of gaps, vague assumptions, and even logical inconsistencies and contradictions which remain uninvestigated by the resident because their investigation is not seen as a relevant pursuit. Resocialisation cannot normally be accomplished by the methods of Thomas Aquinas.

Thirdly, the residents' subjective reality, particularly that imbibed in childhood, contains normative and affective as well as cognitive components. These tacit understandings are invested with piety, and not only do residents normally see it as irrelevant to examine them critically, but they may also be reluctant to conduct such an investigation and recoil distressed from the results.

Finally, and perhaps most importantly for psychiatric practice, it is not the case that everyday knowledge – contradictory and less-than-comprehensive as it is – will capitulate meekly in the face of the rival interpretations of expert knowledge once a confrontation has been forced. If it becomes a relevant pursuit to do so, and if the residents' affective commitment to their contested subjective reality is sufficiently strong, then they are perfectly capable of reconciling apparent contradictions, elaborating the everyday knowledge base to cover apparent gaps and inadequacies, all from within the existing everyday knowledge base, and so rebutting to their own satisfaction the competing expert interpretation.

This brief analysis of the sponge-like conservatism of subjective reality will be no news to psychotherapists, school-teachers, evangelical Christians and others engaged in secondary socialisation, but it does at least set out the problem that therapeutic community practitioners face in constructing an alternative reality for residents.

So far we have emphasised the resistance of everyday knowledge to overthrow and replacement, though of course shifts in what Schutz calls the 'accent reality' can and do occur. However, for the disintegration of the massive reality of childhood to occur spontaneously and unassisted will normally require some severe, prior, biographical disruption; Schutz instances a war hero returning to his old job as a cigar clerk and finding that his war experiences lead him to look upon his old social world with an estranged and leery eye (Schutz, 1964b).

Assisted resocialisation, reality construction in the service of therapy, must employ specific pedagogic techniques. Many of these techniques aim at a similar biographical disjunction to that experienced by the homecoming cigar clerk: the removal of a child to a new social environment remote from family and friends, the prohibition of all contacts between the ex-junkie and his old acquaintances on the outside, the drawing of 'contrast sets' (Smith, 1978) by psychiatric patients contrasting their old 'unreal' social relationships on the outside with the new warm relationships they have struck up in the therapeutic community. In those communities oriented to rehabilitation as well as treatment, this contrast with, and implicit derogation of, the residents' old social world may be a source of problems once discharge looms near. But in the early stages of treatment at least, the communities are not concerned to assimilate the new social world of the treatment setting to the old one, but rather to replace it. In the case of some agencies of resocialisation, notably religious sects such as the Moonies, this displacement and disvaluation of the old social world of the convert has become a source of public controversy, and in a diluted form represents something of an ethical dilemma for therapists in at least some therapeutic communities.

The new subjective reality of the resident will be comprehensive in its coverage; it will contain not just new interpretative schemes, but many understandings that are simply tacit, and even some taboos that are unthinkingly absorbed. Understandings may be tacit because the degree of clarity, elaborateness, or specificity of application of the interpretation may not be required to be very great: it may not be a relevant pursuit for residents to probe the clarity, or whatever, of a given interpretation; the degree of clarity required of an understanding will be that degree required by the resident's purpose at hand.

A crucial aspect of the new subjective reality of the therapeutic community is the vocabulary of its expression. Indeed, the newly learned vocabulary of motives, feeling states and descriptions *constitutes* that subjective reality, since all thought is conceptual, that is, verbal. Reality construction in the therapeutic community involves imbibing (and possibly repeating) a series of accounts – accounts of the community social structure, accounts of the process of therapy, accounts of residents' difficulties, and so on. In the process of learning, those accounts, provided they are not opposed or contradicted by alternative accounts from other sources such as a resident counter-culture, take on the appearance of objective fact – they become the reality of the situation they seek to describe. To resurrect a much-used trope, the new resident is like a stranger in a foreign land who at first struggles to master everyday phrases and labours to translate everything into his native tongue, but eventually that foreign language supplants the native tongue, becomes the language of thought and dreams, and translation is no longer necessary.

The centrality of reality construction in therapeutic community practice, and its problematic character, should both by now be evident; the remainder of this chapter will be concerned with the different methods by which communities attempt reality construction. We shall begin by contrasting the methods adopted by two halfway houses, Ashley and Beeches.

Reality confrontation and instrumentalism – the contrasting cases of Ashley and Beeches

The social construction, or reconstruction, of subjective reality proceeds piecemeal, not suddenly and all at once: particular perceptions of particular events, tasks, or relationships are altered and by a process of cumulation these individual and situated redefinitions may result in the gradual reconstruction of subjective reality. So our interest in methods of reality construction becomes an interest in the methods of *redefining* particular events, and readers should now find our earlier statement – that redefinition is the motor of therapy – more intelligible, alongside our earlier definition of therapeutic work as a cognitive activity which can transform any mundane event in the community by *redefining* that event in the light of some therapeutic paradigm.

The great divide in communities' methods of redefinition lies between those communities which emphasise reality confrontation and those which emphasise instrumentalism. Rather than reiterate our earlier definitions of these terms we will illustrate the divide by an extended discussion of two halfway houses of similar size, Ashley and Beeches, run by the same charitable trust and with similar resident groups of disturbed adolescents (see the descriptions of the houses in Chapter 2). These two similarly circumstanced communities adopted sharply contrasting, almost antithetical, approaches to therapy. Ashley emphasised reality confrontation and Beeches emphasised instrumentalism.

Ashley House

Staff did not normally seek to instruct, oversee and control the performance of tasks by residents but only to monitor and, subsequently, to criticise or praise resident behaviour from the standpoint of the degree of responsibility and independence that was shown. Resident task performance was judged less from the standpoint of satisfactory task completion than from an observed willingness and ability to work independently. Residents who performed poorly in the morning workgroup could expect to be confronted about their irresponsible 'skiving' in the subsequent coffee group. Likewise, residents who slept through workgroup were not routed out of bed but were allowed to slumber on; inadequate resident task performance was not an occasion for immediate staff intervention to ensure task completion, rather resident non-participation was made the topic for subsequent redefinition:

> Coffee group. Dickie had failed to get up for workgroup. Neil (deliberately?) under-reacted to this. Dickie volunteered that he do his cleaning after the coffee group. Later in the group we were discussing the need for a volunteer to help shift the three-piece suite that was being donated to the house. Betty said she would go and Dickie also offered. Neil said it was no good Dickie volunteering because he never did what he said he'd do. Dickie disputed that he was irresponsible: he said he'd throw Neil's words back at him. Neil said he wasn't interested in the future but in the present.

It will be realised that the staff's refusal to occupy a supervisory role ensured a ready flow of topical material for redefinition, especially in respect of new residents used to closely supervised institutional regimes.

Relatedly, staff at Ashley did not see disruptions and quarrels as necessarily requiring an intervention to ensure the smooth running of the house. Staff were prepared to tolerate a degree of disruption in the expectation that the residents themselves would take the initiative in resolving the problem. Late-night disturbances in the bedrooms, for example, were often left to be suppressed by the weight of public opinion. This should not be viewed as a *laissez-faire* attitude; these disruptions were in fact the subjects of a good deal of staff activity: staff would raise the disruption at a coffee group or at the weekly community meeting as a topic for discussion, they would urge on the residents the need for the residents themselves to find a solution, and they would reward with praise all successful efforts. In effect, staff were prepared to allow rather more unruly behaviour in the house than in most institutions because tolerance of that disruption was part of a conscious staff strategy to manipulate the running of the house by indirect means, by the orchestration of a greater individual and collective responsibility among residents. Consider the staff role in the following incident, in which a resident who had a fetish for girls' nightdresses was caught redhanded by a resident with a violent temper:

> Workgroup. Frank (staff) cleaned the lounge and I cleaned the office. We both propped our doors open so that we could monitor the doings of the residents. ... Betty caught Eric going into her room twice: neither I nor Frank moved to intervene although I'm sure, like me, he heard Betty raising her voice (but not screaming abuse). I'm sure, like me, Frank thought it would be best if Betty resolved the situation for herself (I congratulated Betty on her handling of the situation in the coffee group).

By minimising the external regulation (rules, supervision) of residents' behaviour staff aimed to provide a social environment which would reproduce those difficulties with social relationships which the residents had encountered on the outside and which would also reproduce those inappropriate ways of handling such relationships that had possibly led to referral to the house in the first place. By presenting the house as a locale where the resident could try out alternative and more appropriate patterns of behaviour, by disvaluing inappropriate behaviour, by mobilising collective pressure to undertake such experiments, and by rewarding attempts to do so, staff sought to replace external regulation by self regulation.

The experimentation with, and adoption of, new patterns of resident behaviour was often referred to as 'using the house':

> . . . There was some discussion of Dougal coming back to the house in tears on Saturday night. I reminded him that last week he'd said he found it hard to talk about his problems, he bottled it all up 'til it exploded – is that what would happen this time? He was given time to talk. Frank (staff) eventually said that if Dougal felt he couldn't talk in a group, mebbe he should think about talking one-to-one with his counsellor, or mebbe with just a few people he felt he wanted to talk to. Frank said he thought that Dougal was mebbe at the point where he might be leaving: he'd settled well into the house and performed all the house tasks quite well, but now he was at the point where he had to start *using the house* to sort himself out. Did Dougal remember he talked before about his life going round in circles? Things would go well for a time and then things would build up and he'd have to start all over again? This was his chance to break out of the circle, but lots of people failed to make use of the chance and left the house.

Exhortations to 'use the house' might well extend to advocacy of specific lines of action, such as telling a resident to talk to people next time he felt depressed rather than going out and sniffing glue, but this did not extend to leading residents along particular pathways. The staff role in these circumstances was described as 'giving support' or 'sharing'. For example, staff might share with a resident who was starting a job their own earlier difficulties about developing working habits, rising early, and so on. But such sharing was not accompanied by any more direct staff intervention: staff might share their experiences about the difficulty of early rising, but it was the resident's responsibility to get up on time.

Encouragement of behavioural change also occurred through staff emphasising the volitional character of behaviour. For example, staff would deny they decided to give a resident notice to quit, claiming that the resident 'decided' to quit when she hit another resident and broke the 'no violence' rule. More important still in developing this volitional perspective, and making residents aware of alternative avenues of conduct, was the staff practice of drawing residents' attention to their current conduct in 'the here and now': the reality that staff sought to reflect back to residents was the immediate reality. The following example, taken from the staff 'feedback/history book' designed to acquaint off-duty staff with recent events, is a staff member's account of his attempts to get Dickie to look at 'the here and now' on the occasion that Dickie was demanding the return of his medication from the house drugs cabinet so that he could 'block off' on drugs and booze. Note that whereas the novice staff member (Bloor) made the mistake of listening to Dickie's grievances, the author of the account repeatedly drew the resident's attention to the current situation (he'd got the staff member out of bed, etc.) and tried to suggest that the house offered Dickie the chance to work through his projective anger:

> Dickie – things seem to be coming to a head re all anger and frustration over various issues over the last week. . . . Went out in the evening, initially with Ellen. Later woke me up around 12.45 a.m. demanding his tablets (belonging to him 'by law'). Said he'd break down office door, etc. if I refused, which I did, then threatened to make me the 201st murder in Britain (the average being 200/year!). Obviously fairly pissed up – said he was pissed off because he'd not been able to get any drugs in town and wanted his tablets. *I came back with the here and now stuff*:- you've just woken me up, I'm not a 24-hour chemist, etc. – also that I'd phone police if he started breaking the place up. Mick joined us and ended up having a fairly long conversation with Dickie running through his repertoire of grievances against the house, HQ, the staff, the other residents, rules, hypocrisy, etc. *I tried to keep it to him abusing me now.* Dickie got onto a legal tack and said he'd ring police and get their opinion and if no joy – break down office door. We did a few more circles of conversation including it being okay for him to use this place to work through his anger and feelings, etc. – i.e. his agreement on coming here. Dickie kept to his decision and I went to bed. This morning, I find the office door pushed in but no other damage – guess Dickie had cornered himself into doing something.

This 'here and now' reality confrontation and the promotion of different options for resident behaviour served to emphasise behavioural change rather than insight into past difficulties. It was not that staff devalued the development of 'insight' in the psychotherapeutic sense of the word, but its value was seen as dependent on its association with the learning of new patterns of behaviour. When a staff member commented that a resident who broke the law to outrage her parents was actually allowing her parents to dominate her, the warden of the house commented that it was crucial that residents see *and act* on that.

Related to the staff's refusal of a supervisory role and tolerance of disruption was the elaborate presentation of the house as different from an 'institution' and repudiation by staff of a 'caring' role. Staff often employed contrast sets to differentiate their practices from those of other agencies with which the resident had previously been in contact: residents who forgot to collect their medication were not chased up by staff – 'this isn't a hospital'; residents who wanted house equipment, like a record-player, locked away to prevent vandalism were told that that was 'an institutional solution' to the vandalism problem. Staff reactions to deviant resident behaviour would extend beyond the tolerance of disruption, described earlier, to studied under-reaction. The staff response to resident para-suicide was an exemplar of such deliberate under-reaction. At one point during Bloor's fieldwork period a resident took an overdose and fellow residents informed the staff member on overnight duty. He told her that she'd need to go to the hospital to get pumped out but he wasn't going to take her in his car and he was really 'pissed off' with her. Staff believed that para-suicides, hysteria, and the like, were indirect messages of disturbance and their under-reaction was often accompanied by specific requests to residents to communicate their feelings in a more direct way. On the morning after the overdose the same staff member told the resident that he was fed-up with her 'late night games' and she'd have to learn to talk about what was 'bugging' her.

Parenthetically, the disavowal of responsibility for para-suicides carries little danger. As in the reported case, fellow-residents can be relied on to arrange emergency treatment and the staff posture minimises the danger of an epidemic of attention-seeking para-suicides. Of course, staff were prepared to drop this posture in genuine life-or-death circumstances.

The repudiation of a caring staff role was related to the staff preference for 'honest' relations with residents. Staff were critical of other institutions and agencies, believing that they often minimised residents' problems, stressed residents' virtues rather than their failings, and were over-optimistic about residents' prospects. Staff could be observed, on occasion, to walk out of groups in exasperation, to tell particular residents they were heartily sick of them and wished they'd clear off back to where they came from, to refuse to cook a meal for an uncooperative resident, and so on. This emphasis on honest relations permitted staff to adopt a self-actualising role in the house, to behave in ways which were an expression of their sense of self, instead of being required to rein it in. This self-actualising role could be a partial guide to staff practice ('doing what felt right' as one staff member was fond of putting it) and a source of considerable job satisfaction.

A wide range of styles of confrontation could be heard at Ashley, including very gentle and ironical reflection of the resident's conduct as in the following instance:

> Betty had over-reacted to Ellen's use of Mary's record player (in Betty's care while Mary is on remand) when Betty wasn't there – she was being very loud and abusive, both at the time of the incident and in recapitulating the matter in the coffee group. Neil and Nick (both staff) reacted with humour to Betty's outbursts, while putting across the message that Betty's behaviour was a repetition of a time-worn pattern. Betty herself began to punctuate her abuse with smiles and humorously extravagant threats: the message had got across to her through Neil's and Nick's ironical treatment of her rather than through direct confrontation.

Finally, a sense of collective responsibility could be fostered by mundane and matter-of-fact remarks and activities by staff which might have little individual influence but taken together helped to maintain a culture in the house which incoming residents naturally and unthinkingly assimilated – a culture in which various aspects of the staff role were diffused among the residents, and the residents had wide individual and collective responsibilities. For example, threats of violence might lead, not to staff sanctions against the resident making the threats, but to staff members asking all residents at the coffee group how *they* felt about threats of violence being uttered in the house. Even a staff-member's casual remark while watching the television one evening, 'I'll put the kettle on if someone else will make the tea', can serve to reinforce this culture of shared responsibilities.

Beeches House

The rationale of the staff approach at Beeches was that of legislating for change: by creating an elaborate social structure and by overseeing resident performance within that environment staff sought to create new patterns of resident behaviour by regulation and repetition; by the progressive movement of residents through a hierarchy of statuses within the house structure staff sought to preserve residents' newly learned behaviour patterns whilst progressively withdrawing regulatory control and staff supervision so that residents might accomplish a gradual transformation to independence.

There was an extensive programme of activities – domestic, social and educational – in which every activity could be seen as a potential learning situation with skills to be mastered and attitudes to be inculcated. Staff supervised, participated in, planned and monitored these activities. The programme of activities occurred alongside a highly articulated hierarchy of statuses with associated privileges and responsibilities. Initially, new residents found themselves in a highly structured environment, subject to restrictive rules and expectations, albeit with the right to participate equally in the formally democratic daily and weekly meetings. Satisfactory performance in the programme led to a resident progressing up the status hierarchy, and the newly gained rights and privileges of more senior status (later bedtime, part-time work experience, and so on) were themselves thought to be a preparation for independence.

The structure simultaneously provided the security of clear expectations and boundaries (listed procedures, detailed rules, specified sanctions) and provided new and demarcated roles. The structure was thought to maximise the chance of successful assumption of new roles by providing templates for role performance. Residents serving their turn on the dinner preparation rota, for example, were expected to follow specially prepared, near-exhaustively specified recipes and to learn their particular recipes (with staff help and supervision) before embarking on new menus.

In effect the house structure itself was conceived as an agency of therapy – motivating, instructing and rewarding behavioural change. Much of the therapeutic work of the staff centred around their servicing or maintaining that structure as an agency of therapy. This structure-maintenance aspect of staff work can be seen in the following extended fieldnote reporting one of the daily (morning) meetings:

Morning meeting. Taken by Lisa. I found Lisa's performance really impressive in the meeting in the way she worked to reconstitute a sense of the structure of the house during the meeting.

Thus she briefly listed Tim's sins of the last 24 hours culminating in his being late back last night, cutting through various deflecting chatter from Tim about wanting to be a lorry driver. She stressed that Tim had only just been given 'trusted resident status' two days ago, and Tim had not shown that he could be trusted, so his trusted resident status was being withdrawn for a fortnight (i.e. he would not be allowed out of the house on his own).

Then she raised the issue of Sheila being an hour late back last night and the police having to be called. She reminded Sheila that she was on her last chance in the house and that everyone had wanted Ivor to leave because his frequent abscondings had caused the police to be called.

She passed over Sheila's nocturnal activities, merely asking who she'd been with ('on my own') and commenting that she must have inflicted the love bites on her neck with a straw. She concentrated on the matter of what action should be taken. Sheila should be on evening house restriction, but for how long? The residents were asked to comment in turn: Sheila thought she should only be on the restriction for a week, but the majority thought that it should be a fortnight to parallel Tim's position . . .

She got Larry into the morning meeting (as Larry would be on work experience that afternoon he was excused the morning meeting) in order to discuss the fight (which had occurred that morning). . . . Lisa then led off with her understanding of how the fight had occurred (Terry was sore at Larry because he hadn't taken his turn at cleaning the bedroom, told Larry to do it, Larry refused and swore at Terry). Lisa asked if this was correct – yes. She then carefully asked Terry whether he'd planned to hit Larry before he went into the Resource Room to get him to clean the bedroom. No, it wasn't planned violence. The importance of this, well understood by the residents, is that the house-rules strictly forbid planned violence and Terry is already on a 'violence warning'. Lisa accepted that it wasn't planned and so merely extended Terry's violence warning by one week.

Next she turned to Larry. She asked if the residents knew what 'provoking' meant – they did. She said Larry had provoked

> Terry. Tony said it took two to make a fight. Larry said he hadn't been fighting: Terry said Larry had hit him on the nose. Others expressed their opinion. Lisa took the consensus and put Larry on a one-week violence warning. She asked if the rota that Larry and Terry had worked out for cleaning their room wasn't working anymore. No it wasn't. Tony said that Terry got told off by the staff for not doing the room but the staff never told off Larry when he didn't do the room. Lisa replied that staff didn't expect to have to tell senior residents to do this and do that: senior residents were expected to be able to make their own decisions and do tasks without supervision. She disposed of Larry's argument that he hadn't had time to do the room by taking Larry through the things he had done since he'd got up to show how he could have organised his time to do the room. She suggested that the old rota be resurrected. Agreed.

Various facets of staff structure maintenance are evident in Lisa's performance. Note in the first place how events in the house such as the fight are related to the house structure: Lisa reconstitutes the house structure for residents as a framework within which events such as the Larry-Terry fight are to be seen and judged, for example, by her allusions to Larry's responsibilities as a senior resident and by her proposal for a structural resolution of the Larry-Terry dispute (a return to the old cleaning rota). In speaking of the staff presentation to residents of the house structure as a 'framework', we imply more than simply a perspective from which events in the house can be viewed, rather we refer to the presentation of the house structure as the accent or paramount reality of the residents' lives. By the repetitive relation of events to the house structure Lisa and her colleagues sought to present the structure as more than just a particular alternative scheme of interpretation but rather as *the* scheme of interpretation which the residents themselves would eventually unthinkingly adopt, endorse and inhabit in their daily lives. Staff activities sought to constitute the house structure as a taken-for-granted social reality. Note here that there was no dispute or debate about whether Sheila should be on evening house restriction, but only about the length of the period for which the restriction should extend: Lisa and residents alike (including Sheila herself) tacitly endorsed the view that some sanction was required.

Also relevant here is Lisa's successful invitation to residents to participate in the social reality which she is presenting. The subjective reality of the house structure is given further endorsement by residents in, for example, their participation in the debate over the 'correct' sanction for Sheila's nocturnal episode.

One final point about staff structure maintenance: the house structure was a therapeutic instrument to be used selectively and flexibly. Of course, the house structure was itself discriminatory in that it discriminated between different statuses ('trusted' resident, 'senior' resident, etc.), but even this discriminatory structure was only creatively and selectively applied. In the present instance Terry was already on an unexpired two-week 'violence warning' for previous violence and the normal response to a repetition of violence in this period would be to place the resident on a 'contract', where any further repetition would lead to the resident's suspension from the house. Lisa's careful delimination of Terry's behaviour as unplanned violence rather than planned violence served to mitigate the offence in the eyes of the meeting and allowed her merely to extend Terry's violence warning rather than put Terry on a contract, which would have left him just one false step away from suspension from the house.

The staff conceived of the house structure as an agency of therapy whose effectiveness would depend on its repetitious presentation as a taken-for-granted reality: if Tina refused to go to 'recreation' on a Friday afternoon she must simply be told that she had do recreation as it was part of the 'programme'. But staff were nevertheless aware that such repetition must be selective and not ritualistic, the selection depending on staff judgments, and care was usually taken, as in the present instance, to present staff behaviour to residents as being consistent with the house structure.

Up to now we have been concerned with those aspects of structure maintenance at Beeches that relate to the repair and repetitive representation of the elaborate status hierarchy of the house (with attendant rights and obligations) as the paramount or accented social reality of the house: any disregard for that reality (such as Sheila's late arrival home, or Terry and Larry's attempt to settle a dispute with their fists rather than through formal discussion and regulation) demanded maintenance work by staff to repair the breach and reassert the house structure. But there is another, analytically distinct, aspect of staff structure maintenance, namely the direct supervision of resident task performance within the house structure. The structure is maintained by overseeing and directing resident activities in conformity with the house structure.

Two staff were normally assigned to the morning workgroup, one of whom was meant to participate in the cleaning work in a particular 'workgroup area', such as the kitchen, while the other was meant to assume a more distinctly supervisory role moving about the house. Staff work included the 'clocking' of late arrivals to be assigned equivalent 'make-up time' at the weekends, ensuring that all the listed cleaning tasks were done and done correctly, ensuring that there was no skiving off, sorting out any disruptions or administrative problems (like finding the missing oven cleaner), and accompanying the resident chairperson on his or her daily inspection of the house checking on the performance of those in the workgroup.

We have already referred (in Chapter 2) to the way in which Beeches staff work was itself regulated by the detailed staff 'operations manual'. The manual illustrates the pervasiveness of the planning orientation to staff work. Staff sought to shape and to anticipate events rather than react to them: staff were to act with one voice, the house structure was to be maintained as a flexible instrument, and residents were to be 'programmed' towards behavioural change. Consider these notes on a staff meeting discussing the imminent return of Roger, a resident who had absconded:

> Lisa asked Jean (Roger's counsellor) to comment on what she thought the staff response to Roger should be on his return. Jean said it would be important to counter Roger's fantasies by getting him to set realistic immediate goals: staff should emphasise immediate goals that he could work towards (e.g. getting a later weekend bedtime by not having any weekend make-up time to do, saving enough money to go to the youth club next week, etc.). Lisa amplified this by saying perhaps we could elicit from Roger something that he would like to do in the immediate future (like a train-trip [to a neighbouring city] or visit to the local radio station): this could be a reward for two weeks good behaviour in the house. Lisa said that studies showed that reinforcement was always more effective if the subject chose his own reward.

Various members of the Beeches staff had been influenced by the principles of psycho-education, an approach to therapy originating in Canada. Integrating the work of Piaget and Erikson, psycho-education sees adolescent behavioural and personality problems as arising out of faulty 'epigenetic' development, out of a failure to proceed successfully through all the various stages of normal child development. The practice of psycho-education entails the very detailed programming of the adolescent's activities by the therapeutic team in order to literally re-educate the adolescent by reproducing in prescribed conduct the various phases of child development in a manner that is no longer faulty and cumulatively damaging (see Gauthier, 1980).

Despite this intellectual influence, Beeches staff were uncertain about the feasibility of pursuing a psycho-education approach in residential treatment settings because of the very high staff in-put that psycho-education required. The overall orientation of the staff could more accurately be described as educative, rather than psycho-educative, in that the amount of planning of resident activities might broadly parallel the lesson-planning entailed in modern team teaching methods. However, one staff member did conduct a regular ceramics class which explicitly incorporated psycho-education programming principles (see Bloor, 1984, pp. 58–62).

Aside from the programming of resident activities, staff also felt that the inculcation of a planning orientation in residents would greatly increase the residents' chances of successful task completion and so break the discouraging 'failure cycle' which was thought to beset residents; thus a planning orientation on the part of staff might carry over into a planning orientation among residents by a kind of cultural osmosis. Staff thus sought to encourage planning by residents on appropriate occasions – witness Bloor's Sunday afternoon endeavours below:

> I spent part of the afternoon helping two residents to lay a carpet in their bedroom. When Lisa (staff) asked me to do it the other day she said that we could make a 'project' out of it, by which I took her to mean that I should approach the job with the explicit intention of ensuring that Larry and Terry should derive some therapeutic benefit from the job: the job was more than just laying a carpet.
>
> I tried to introduce an element of planning into the job, especially since I knew that one of the reasons that Terry sometimes fails at tasks he sets himself is that he will leap into the job without considering what is entailed. I was only partially successful in this: I did get them to think about what furniture should be moved out of the room first . . . but I had great

> difficulty explaining to them the principle of using the old carpet as a template...

It will already be evident that a good deal of staff planning and staff structure maintenance was aimed at the avoidance of disruption, the successful completion of resident tasks, the smooth running of community activities, and so on. And indeed, although Beeches staff could be seen to engage in reality confrontation on occasion, for the most part they avoided such disruptive interventions. Instead, Beeches staff sought to achieve therapeutic goals instrumentally, the success of a staff intervention perhaps depending on the staff goal remaining hidden from the resident and so circumventing possible resident opposition – see, for example, two fieldwork extracts concerning Bloor's failures and successes in intervening with Roger, a particularly dreamy and Walter Mitty-ish resident:

> Told Lisa I was at a loss as to how to handle Roger. I found I had to be very direct to get through to him – humour and allusion are lost on Roger – but directness provoked a tough-guy response ('Get *lost*, I'm not doing *that* [slams door]). Lisa suggested that I preface all my interventions with the 'Listen technique' – 'Listen Roger, I need to have a serious talk with you...'

And:

> I had Roger by myself for education. He was both reluctant to work and reluctant to do the type of work specified in his education programme. Adopted the approach that Lisa had previously suggested of prefacing my remarks with 'Listen Roger, we need to have a serious talk ...' and then, having got his attention, making my point. Worked like a charm. In the morning work group I'd had similar success with Roger using this approach.

Recognising that different styles of intervention would be differentially effective in different circumstances and for different residents, staff attempted to distinguish six different 'categories' of interventions – informative, prescriptive, confrontative, catalytic, cathartic, and supportive – and would list the category or categories of intervention approved for each resident in an 'intervention book'.

That the routine social life of the house can itself be of therapeutic import is widely recognised. At Beeches such benign routines were thought to have a value in various ways – as a release from the pressures of therapeutic community life, in giving a sense of security to an adolescent resident group through their repetitious familiarity, and in giving adolescents an opportunity to mix socially with persons outside their peer group:

> Len (staff) and I had a two-a-side game of football with Harry and Kevin. Len not above a little dexterous fouling and gamesmanship, not above persuading Harry to fetch the ball after he (Len) had booted it next door. Later on Len lost 20p to Terry at snooker – more horseplay in the office later when he paid Terry in pennies. Finally, Len, Harry and I sat and watched *Match of the Day*, commenting intermittently on the game, the players, etc. All these events had a natural quality: there was no *overt* therapeutic content to what Len did and said. Len was not being one of the boys but more father-like – no descent to the level of swearing or lewdity, merely a mature adult offering adolescents the opportunity to interact with him in a relaxed, friendly, but adult manner.

Contrasts and similarities between the two houses

That reality confrontation and instrumentalism are indeed contrasting approaches can be verified by taking some field of resident activity common to both houses and examining the respective approaches. Several such fields of activity might be looked at in this way; here we choose to examine differences in therapeutic work respecting meal preparation (elsewhere, Bloor, 1986, has contrasted the approaches to house cleaning).

In both houses communal meals were prepared on a rota basis, but there the similarity ended. At Beeches, cooking was seen as an opportunity for residents to 'break the failure cycle' by successfully preparing a sometimes elaborate evening meal: to ensure success there were specially prepared recipes which provided instructions at a far more detailed level than any cookery book, and there was also close supervision from staff; the same residents would repeat the same menu for several weeks until it was learned by repetition; staff and residents were scrupulous in thanking the cooks and praising good work. At Ashley, cooking was seen as an opportunity for residents to be led towards taking on more responsibility for their actions: although staff played their part on the rota, they would not supervise the cooking or shopping, and were prepared to tolerate poor task performance to the extent of no meal being served at all, in order that irresponsibility be brought home to erring residents (those who refused to cook could expect to be confronted by aggrieved fellow-residents). In one house meal preparation was a particular focus for staff planning and supervision, in the other house meal-preparation was an area of activity where staff made a particular effort to withdraw from any supervisory role.

Having established, we hope, that these two approaches to therapy, despite being applied in similar institutions in respect of similar client groups, were indeed almost diametrically opposed, it is necessary to introduce a few caveats. In the first place, it should be recognised that principles of therapy that seemed sharply contrasting at an abstract level could sometimes be quite similar in their practical applications. Consider how, below, the concern at Ashley for 'honest' relations with residents might have very similar effects to the use at Beeches of formal 'contracts' to hold erring residents to more acceptable behaviour:

> In the afternoon staff meeting I asked Neil what should be done about Dougal (who had absconded) if he came back today or tomorrow . . . Neil said that Frank (absent) had suggested that we ask Dougal to agree to abide by certain limits on his behaviour for a certain period of time, e.g. in by 11 o'clock each night, and in at mealtimes. I asked if this should be tied to the production of a report to his probation officer from the house in respect of his court case coming up next month, like a 'contract'. Neil said that, for himself, he would prefer to put it that the house would be writing an honest report and its content would naturally depend on Dougal's behaviour – he said that was almost the same, but there was a difference. Did I see it?

In the second place, it must be recognised that the differences we have described were differences of emphasis. Instances of benign routine, similar to those at Beeches, could also be found at Ashley, although routine at Ashley was not seen to promote therapy directly but rather to provide a context for therapy. More importantly, reality confrontation and instrumentalism were observable in both communities.

Instances of reality confrontation could be seen at Beeches, although never with the aims of disrupting routine or provoking dissent. Most frequently, reality confrontation could be observed in an 'open discussion' section of the weekly community meeting, where it fitted well with the reflective purpose of the meeting, but it could also sometimes be heard in the promotion of compliance and maintenance of the house structure.

Similarly, some of the reality confrontation at Ashley might actually be described as being instrumental in character, since the main subject of the confrontation was to engineer a counter-reaction from the resident that could itself be turned to therapeutic account. Note, for example, Dave's attempts to engineer a cathartic run-in between Victor and an authority figure:

> Victor (resident) . . . was down on the rota today for washing up (which includes laying the tables). Dave (staff), who was cooking, had already reminded Victor once to lay up. When Dave came to serve up the food he found that Victor hadn't done the job properly. Dave stormed out of the dining room and gave Victor an earful. I and the rest of the community (helping ourselves to food) could hear Dave yelling at Victor to stop arsing about, and to pull his weight, to get himself together or move out, not to bother eating Dave's cooking if he wouldn't pull his weight, etc.

Later:

> He told me that he felt that Victor needed him to come the authoritative father: Victor needed to work out his relationships with authority. He went on to say (jokingly) that he sometimes felt that all he needed to do in the house was to breeze around bawling people out and generally throw his weight about.

And it will not have escaped the attention of alert readers that the orchestration of events practised by Ashley staff has itself instrumental undertones, even though the object being so instrumentally sought is likely to be the reflection of an erring resident's conduct back to him or her by fellow community members.

At the risk of appearing paradoxical we can state that Ashley staff often sought reality confrontation by instrumental means, and that Beeches staff often used reality confrontation as a means of instrumental resocialisation. Furthermore, both houses made use of both approaches and the distinction we are making between them is one of relative emphasis, albeit a considerable one. If we were to represent a purely reality-confronting approach and a purely instrumental approach as the two poles of a continuum, then Ashley would be close to the former, and Beeches to the latter.

A final caveat: comparisons which dwell exclusively on contrasting practices are clearly selective and distorting. There was one strong parallel in practice between the two houses and that was the centrality of monitoring or surveillance in both communities. The monitoring work of the staff extended well beyond the bounds of the formal programme. This similarity in the pervasiveness of monitoring, whereby staff surveillance could potentially extend into every corner of resident life, was not always matched by a similarity of form. The supervisory role and the quasi-parental position of the staff at Beeches naturally promoted overt surveillance, whilst the withdrawal of Ashley staff from a supervisory role coupled with attempts to orchestrate behaviour in the community led more frequently to covert surveillance: one staff member remarked that the reason he so frequently did his laundry whilst on the overnight shift lay in the natural opportunity it provided him for observational forays between the office and the laundry area in the kitchen.

The centrality of monitoring in both houses stemmed from the fact that monitoring was a prerequisite of all intervention, be it reality confrontation or programming: all staff intervention depended on prior monitoring and reflectivity, on prior redefinition of a mundane event as a necessary or an appropriate occasion for intervention. For the same reason monitoring was a collective staff project. Staff needed to share monitored information on residents because of the need for collaborative and/or consistent staff action, and because of the need to develop a joint case-picture of a resident. Monitoring is a prerequisite for cumulative therapeutic work, building on previous information to develop progressively the resident's abilities.

The other communities

It remains for us now to consider the relative position of the other communities in the study. Considerations of space preclude further descriptions in the same amount of detail as we supplied for Ashley and Beeches. We can only assert similarities, concentrating our attention on distinguishing and contrasting features of particular approaches to therapy.

The day hospital

We can note various parallels between practice in the day hospital and at Ashley. There was a parallel tolerance of disruptive 'acting out' behaviour by patients, so that at the day hospital, too, patients repeated those difficulties they had experienced in the wider society. There was a parallel monitoring of such acting out and repeated reality confrontation to direct the subject's gaze to his or her unacceptable behaviour. Just as Ashley residents were invited or exhorted to 'use the house' to try out new and non-pathogenic ways of relating to others, so also at the day hospital patients were called upon to 'use the groups'. Likewise, the volitional character of behaviour was emphasised by a similar Gestalt emphasis on behaviour in the 'here and now'. And again, the nursing staff sought to distance themselves from a traditional hospital nursing role, mixing informally with patients and emphasising their rights and obligations as 'members of the group' rather than as staff members. And finally, day hospital staff were similarly prepared to use reality confrontations instrumentally (recall Dave's denunciation of Victor's table-laying) to orchestrate a cathartic denouement.

Of course, some differences were observable between the day hospital and the Ashley treatment approaches, but most of these were of seemingly minor importance. For example, since only a minority of the day hospital patients were residential (see Chapter 2) the staff had much less opportunity than the Ashley staff to monitor the doings of the patients outside the groups and indeed were largely dependent for their information concerning outside occurrences on self-disclosure or reportage from fellow patients. Perhaps partly as a consequence, day hospital staff directed relatively more reality confrontation/redefinitional work towards the behaviour of patients in the context of the groups themselves – patients' willingness or unwillingness to participate, their readiness to see parallels between other patients' problems and their own, their 'honesty', their 'defensiveness', their posture and demeanour, and so on and so forth. To a greater extent than at Ashley, various aspects of a subject's behaviour within a group therapy session were likely to be a focus for inspection and confrontation in the context of that same session.

Of more importance perhaps was the difference between the day hospital and Ashley in the extent to which the former had been able to penetrate and mobilise the patient culture as a treatment resource. Many and varied are the sociological studies of psychiatric institutions which show patients subverting the aims of those institutions in favour of their own immediate needs and gratifications (Belknap, 1956; Caudill, 1958; Goffman, 1968; Braginsky et al., 1969). And yet therapeutic communities, far from acquiescing in this subcultural subversion of the formal treatment programme, seek to mobilise the patient culture as a treatment resource. The problematic relationship between the day hospital's formal treatment programme and the patient culture has been fully reported elsewhere (Bloor, 1980b; Bloor, 1981) but we may briefly summarise the findings here.

As at Ashley, staff at the day hospital expected a good deal of the work of reality confrontation to be conducted by fellow-patients. Such peer confrontations took place outside, as well as inside, the formal groups:

> In the pub Greta asked Harry what he had meant by saying (earlier) that he had things to say to her. Harry at first refused to elaborate in that context, saying that she should ask him in the group and then he would certainly tell her. Greta persisted and Harry eventually relented and went into a long discourse on how Greta was too selfless and allowed other people . . . to make too many demands on her and she should think much more about her own needs and be more demanding herself. Greta agreed in principle but said it was impossible in practice – these people really needed her. I joined Harry . . . we countered that if these people were worth anything at all they would certainly understand if Greta told them she couldn't help anybody just now until she'd helped herself, that if Greta was in their position she would certainly understand that, and so on. Greta eventually agreed.

Further, since day hospital staff had less direct access to observe patient behaviour than would be the case in residential settings, staff would urge on patients the importance of free communications and, particularly where patients were meeting socially (and sometimes intimately) outside the groups, they depended on fellow-patients to urge unhappy confidants to 'go public' by telling their secrets to the groups:

> ... Mary (patient) was angry at people who had spoken at the social and been silent in the group. She'd been put in a very difficult position: someone had cried in her arms and made her promise not to tell the group. Still silence. She named three people and one of them ... immediately began to speak.

Day care facilities are extremely easy to default from: the would-be patient defaulter has only to stay away from the facility on the following morning. Since group therapy can be highly stressful, the danger of provoking unacceptably high defaulting rates is a very real one. There is also the danger (well recognised by therapists) that the stresses of treatment may lead some patients to suicidal impulses. At the day hospital it was a convention, encouraged by staff, that fellow-patients provided each other with comfort and support and helped each other to remain in treatment:

> ... This afternoon considerable pressure was put on Dave: he spoke of his feelings of helplessness and depression, his failure to 'work' in the group, and his feeling that he ought to leave the day hospital. [At the end of the afternoon] several staff-members had already left for prior appointments. Edith (staff) said she'd seen Dave glance at the clock several times: now was his chance to end it. His voice breaking, Dave ... said he'd end it alright and rushed out of the room. Edith did nothing to stop him. At Harriet's (patient) bidding, Nick (patient) went after him, caught him up in the toilets, and eventually made him promise to come in again tomorrow. Once before he'd dashed off and his fellow-patients had set off after him: indeed this dashing after bolting patients is a fairly common occurrence – Edith could predict that Dave would be looked after.

On several occasions during Bloor's fieldwork patients would send a delegation (which sometimes, but not always, included a staff member) to call on a defaulting patient at home to persuade them back to the hospital. No patient who had made perfectly clear their determination to quit was subjected to such persuasion, but others had to resort to subterfuge to avoid such house calls: one patient, who had been visited (and recalled) once previously, was thought to be at home but refusing to answer the door, while another secretly left the country.

It will be evident from this account of the therapeutic work that patients conducted at the day hospital that the patient culture had been extensively penetrated. Indeed, the patients showed many of the characteristics of sectarian converts: they peppered their conversations with in-group argot and catchphrases ('How do you feel about that?'), they earnestly continued their group discussions into lunch-breaks and after-hours meetings, they endlessly discussed the behaviour, strengths and foibles of staff members, they fell in love, they fell away from earlier friendships and instead developed intense emotional ties with fellow-patients that transcended every barrier of age and class. However, this penetration of the patient culture was not absolute, as we shall show in Chapter 5.

The concept house

The location of the concept house for addicts on our reality confrontation/instrumentalism continuum is more problematic. In many respects the approach of the concept houses is an accentuation of the instrumentalist approach reported at Beeches – the prohibition of all contact with outsiders in the early stages of residence, the extensive programming of activities (including the residents' leisure hours), the very close supervision of activities and exacting standards of task performance, a hierarchy of statuses with associated rights and obligations, and so on.

Yet in one respect the concept house approach echoes Ashley in its attempt to orchestrate cathartic confrontations between community members. These cathartic confrontations – 'pull-ups', 'haircuts', and the abusive exchanges of the encounter groups – are vividly denunciatory and amount to reality confrontations. In fact Sugarman, writing of the Daytop Village concept house, describes the approach as 'reality therapy ... forcing [the resident] to look objectively at how he acts and the consequences of his actions and demanding that he change behaviour that does not conform to the "Daytop Concept"' (Sugarman, 1974, p. 17). And 'The Philosophy', read out semi-religiously every morning at Fonkert's concept house as well as a Daytop, reads in part: 'until a man confronts himself in the eyes and hearts of his fellows, he is running.'

Is it possible then that we have misrepresented the relationship between reality confrontation and instrumentalism? Far from being poles on a continuum, are they capable of being harmoniously merged? And are the concept houses this kind of synthetic development? We would argue not, and that our original scheme holds good. Whilst at Ashley and the day hospital the reflection back of the subject's conduct was frequently a gentle affair, sometimes ironical, sometimes hesitant in its conclusions, at the concept house reality confrontation was normally denunciatory. These denunciations can be linked to another aspect of the approach of the concept houses, namely their degradation ceremonies – being put 'on the stool' on arrival, the shearing of hair, the exchange of personal clothing for overalls, 'therapeutic measures' such as the requirement to carry a signboard recording one's transgressions, the requirement of public confessions, and so on. Both the degradation ceremonies and the denunciations are aspects of what the staff term 'image-blowing', the forcible stripping away of the addict's favourable self-image. They also serve, as mentioned previously, to orchestrate catharsis. They are also, self-evidently, mechanisms of social control. And finally they are expressions of group solidarity, public occasions where the community can affirm its solidarity by reviling the deviant whose backsliding uncomfortably reminds them of their own potential frailty.

Crucially, these confrontations are not the pivot of therapy, they do not sketch out a situation of resident choice. Recall, in our discussion of Ashley House, Frank's remarks to Dougal on his chance to break out of the circle by resolving to start 'using the house'. In the concept houses denunciations contain no such volitional element, and therapeutic work is not directed towards a climacteric of decision-making. Rather, in the concept house, residents are *told* what they must do: there is no choice to be made; choices ended upon their entry into the community. Residents are not even told, in the early stages of treatment, why they must do things. Fonkert was told, when he looked for explanations, 'Do the community, experience it, explaining and understanding is not so important – that will come later.'

Just as at Beeches, concept house residents are instructed and directed in new patterns of behaviour and these new patterns of behaviour are assimilated into their stock of commonsense knowledge and have a taken-for-granted character. But in contrast to the approach at Beeches, the resident's previous patterns of behaviour are simultaneously disparaged; opposition is not circumvented by skilful intervention ('Listen Roger, I need to have a serious talk with you...') but is met head on by reality confrontation. At the concept house reality confrontation is not a technique of volitional behaviour change, but rather it is the precursor of, and an aid to, the programming of resident behaviour.

In respect of our earlier discussion of the mobilisation of the resident culture, it is important to stress that the concept houses are staffed largely or wholly by ex-addicts. If we add to this an elaborate hierarchy of statuses (see Chapter 2), subject to frequent promotion and demotion reflecting current performance, then no clear cut staff/resident distinction is possible. The concept house, in Sugarman's happy phrase, is 'a boarding school run by the prefects' (Sugarman, 1975, p. 144).

Addicts' social relations are the sociological exemplar of the deviant subculture. But the concept houses provide little seed ground for subcultural growth. Rules prohibit outside contact and even social mixing between residents who knew each other 'on the outside'. All socialising must take place in groups and no sexual pairings are permitted. All residents' doings are closely scrutinised and subject to frequent 'pull-ups' and 'hair cuts'. Leisure is curtailed and tasks are strenuous and demanding. The rewards of conformity are considerable: access is offered to a world of close, warm relationships, characterised, it is claimed, by honesty and social responsibility, superior to the outside society (once more the Utopian connotations); commitment is rewarded by delighted hugs and formal praise (the 'positive haircut'); and the convert's achievements are recited in biographical form at the house meetings as a boost to self esteem.

The absence of subcultural supports for any alternative perspective on events in the house hastens the process described earlier of reality construction through unthinking assimilation. Residents learn the argot of the community; the Dutch house had taken over many terms, untranslated ('haircut', 'space out' and so on), from the American houses. Residents learn, by trial and error, how to behave correctly in the house. In the course of a work group, a new resident tried to arrange something with an expeditor (a senior member of the hierarchy). The expeditor replied that he should do it 'through the structure', that is, he should do it through his immediate superior, the assistant foreman.

Neither the argot, nor the prescriptions for resident behaviour, can unambiguously connote the objects, events, activities, and states of mind to which they refer. Nor can the occasions of their use be exhaustively specified. The social reality of the concept house itself, like other therapeutic communities and like all the social worlds we inhabit, has only that degree of clarity or specificity required by its inhabitants for the purpose at hand. Fonkert sometimes provoked irritation when he asked for clarification of the meaning of some of the house slang. Similarly, no learned prescription is a straightforward template for action and the circumstances of its application can only be provisionally stated.

However, collectivity members – inhabitants of the social world of the concept house – go about their business *as if* their argot communicated their meaning and *as if* the behaviour prescriptions provided templates for action, since they were indeed adequate for their immediate purposes at hand. In assimilating, and successfully using in their turn, the argot and behavioural prescriptions of the concept house, new residents also assimilate osmotically this unexamined (for the moment) sense of the adequate comprehensibility and specificity of their social world. What was on arrival puzzling or even bizarre is eventually taken for granted, even though meticulous enquiry would still reveal residual and unresolvable ambiguity. The resident now shares the social reality of his compeers.

The Camphill community

It is difficult to conceive of a sharper apparent contrast between the pressure cooker of the concept house and the Arcadian tranquillity of a Camphill community. And yet both communities pursue a broadly instrumental approach.

Konig, the founder of the Camphill movement, described 'three essentials' of the Camphill approach (Konig, 1965). The first of these principles is the recognition that within the handicapped child dwells an infinite and eternal spiritual being. The second is the creative power or potential of the co-worker. The third principle comes as something of a surprise: it is . . . 'sociology'! By this Konig referred to a kind of social engineering, creating the correct kind of social environment in which the developmental potential of handicapped and disturbed children could be fulfilled.

At the most general level, this instrumental approach, this manipulation of the child's social relationships and activities, can be seen as paradoxically permissive. Within Camphill the object is not to impose some new pattern of behaviour, nor to convert the child to a new social world, but rather to achieve the social conditions which will allow the spiritual being within the child to achieve its spiritual purpose, to reach the goals that it sought when it incarnated within a handicapped body. The co-worker's task is to remove the external frustrations and ease the inner torments of the handicapped child, so that the child may come to terms with his or her own handicap and find peace in recognising his or her destiny.

The various components of therapy at Camphill communities, such as curative eurythmy and the school, can be seen, at the same level of generality, to effect this permissive instrumentalism. The school curriculum, for example, is held to be so shaped as to facilitate the progressive incarnation of the spirit into the handicapped body, to permit the emergence of a symbiotic relationship between the spirit and its handicapped 'sheath'.

At the level of everyday practice, many instrumental interventions designed to permit this spiritual development may also be experienced as constraints. Thus the children are removed from various possibly harmful external influences (notably the television) but these may be seen by the children as deprivations even while they enjoy the benefits. Consider the case of the moments of silence and bodily stillness that are required both during worship and immediately prior to the midday meal. It is thought to be most beneficial for these children – handicapped, psychotic, hyperkinetic, and otherwise disturbed – to attempt to assume control over their bodies and inclinations. Further, various commentators have remarked upon the extraordinary dignity and tranquillity of the children on these occasions, especially during the religious services (Clarke, 1974, provides a parallel report on the Catholic L'Arche communities). The children, it might be argued, rise to the occasion, but equally the occasion must be provided by the co-workers: the co-workers must plan, monitor, and supervise.

The redefinition of mundane events was not an *explicit* feature of Camphill community activities: a dormitory parent would not tell a child that she was to be dressed in such a way as to gain a sense of rhythmical movement. An instrumental approach to therapy, as we have seen, achieves its object unremarked by the subject. The Camphill approach has affinities with the Geel foster family and much emphasis is placed on the creation of a benign routine, within which the child experiences the security of clear expectations. The task of the co-workers is to maintain this benign routine while simultaneously finding within it the occasions for therapeutic intervention. This is achieved by a frontstage/backstage distinction (see Chapter 5) and by backstage reflection and planning among co-workers, both individually and collectively:

During the coffee break the co-workers discuss taking the children to the beach. There is a problem, though, because the house bus can only take a limited number of children, so certain kids must be left at home. The adults decide who is to go and who is to remain in the house.

GARY: It would be really good for James to go. He hates doing anything in a group so he is a definite.

ULRIKE: Simon need not go. We should tell him and make it sound like a punishment for being so cheeky. Tell him that he was to go but because of his behaviour he no longer will.

It would be superfluous to describe in detail here the work of backstage redefinition and associated intervention (the reader can find a detailed account in McKeganey, 1982). Instead, we will comment on two particular aspects of co-workers' therapeutic work which seemingly stand out by comparison with other communities discussed earlier.

One such aspect of the co-worker's redefinitional work was the attention paid to promoting particular associations of children. It was thought that relations between children with different difficulties could be mutually beneficial – a handicapped child could derive considerable benefit from being given the opportunity of looking after another more handicapped child; Down's Syndrome children, because of their normally affectionate behaviour, were thought to have considerable potential to help the emotionally deprived. At the Camphill community co-workers were able to exercise a considerable degree of control over these associations. Because the co-workers were in loco parentis they could decide who should sit with whom at mealtimes, which children should be taken on house outings, which children should share dormitories, and so on.

Another seemingly unusual feature of the Camphill community, relative to others discussed so far, was the difference between senior and junior co-workers in the content of expressed redefinitions. In all communities there will be many conversations among staff members where the redefinitions employed will be heavily glossed, either because the speaker can appeal to the hearer's understanding to elaborate the meaning of the utterance, or because the public setting, or the onrush of events, only allows an abbreviated comment. The Camphill community was no exception, and exchanges such as that below, about a trampolining child in the gym, could commonly be heard:

> CO-WORKER 1: Don't let her bounce around . . . it's really bad for her . . . makes her really cuckoo.
> CO-WORKER 2: I don't know, I thought it was good for her.
> CO-WORKER 1: I'm not telling you for this time . . . but for others really: it's not good for her.
> CO-WORKER 2: OK, I didn't know. I don't think it used to be.

The instrumental approach to therapy ensures that interventions by co-workers do not disrupt the benign routine of the house and the wider community; indeed many interventions can be seen as protecting this routine against breakdown and disruption. The rhythmic structure of the child's day has already been described in Chapter 2. A similar 'rhythmic structure' shapes the child's year with preparations for, and celebrations of, the great Christian festivals. Weihs has commented as follows:

> It has frequently been remarked upon how profoundly and positively very disturbed children change and improve within weeks of their being admitted to one of the Curative Houses. This is not due to the immediate results of any of the therapies or medicaments applied, but rather to the children's response to the rhythmic-dynamic structure of life in these schools. (Weihs, 1975, p. 104)

These various therapies (curative eurythmy, music therapy, drama therapy, and so on) and the medications (homeopathic and allopathic) prescribed in the regular clinics have been referred to elsewhere and will not be elaborated upon here. But no description of therapeutic relationships at a Camphill community would be complete without some account, no matter how inadequately expressed, of the selfless relations between co-workers and children. Konig termed these relations the second of the 'three essentials' of Camphill. Co-workers give up long hours of sleep to comfort restless, disturbed children; hours in a day will be given up to companionship with a deaf and dumb child. Co-workers must endure and sacrifice in order to give to the handicapped child. In giving, Konig argued, they will also receive, both from the handicapped child and also from a developing inner, spiritual education. And in this giving and receiving there must be no taint of an economic relationship:

> To give and to take is a matter of mutual human relationship; the true relationship goes as soon as wages intervene. Paid service is no service; paid love is no love; paid help has nothing to do with help. (Konig, 1965, p. 151)

Even without Konig's proscription of wage relationships, it will already be obvious to readers that dedicated and self-sacrificing staff members, often sustained by a Utopian collective enthusiasm, are to be found in many communities.

Parkneuk

The approach to therapy at Parkneuk, like that at the Camphill community, was instrumental in character. Of course, as a secular community, there was no conception of therapy as oriented to the reconciliation of the incarnated spirit with its handicapped body. Rather, at the most general level, the object of therapy was to equip the adolescent boarders with sufficient work, domestic, and social skills to allow them to graduate to an adult community for the handicapped like Newton Dee village. The daily tasks of the boarders were planned, monitored, and supervised with a view to inculcating these skills. Consider Tom's remarks about Victor, a withdrawn schizophrenic:

> Tom says Victor has been much worse since his return from the Christmas holidays and he fears they (the co-workers) may have made him worse by losing their tempers with him. They have now instituted a new regime: he is set a task and shown how to do it and then is simply left to complete it in his own time. Today was the first day. Tom had planned out the construction of a welly boot rack for him.
>
> Tom felt my arrival today was fortuitous: I could work on the loft ladder in the workshop and help out Victor if he got in a mess.
>
> Tom felt Victor had responded very well to the new approach. He drew my attention to the fact that immediately before supper Victor had asked Tom 'Have I done enough today?' Tom felt that such work-related conversational initiatives were rarities from Victor – he's usually much more passive.

As at the Camphill community, this instrumental approach was clearly adopted in order to allow therapeutic work to co-exist peacefully with the benign routine of the community, which was in itself adjudged therapeutic in respect of the security and firm expectations it gave to the boarders. Much staff work in fact was devoted to the maintenance and protection of these benign routines, which were naturalistic rather than natural, family-like rather than familial. Reality confrontation, where it did occur, normally had a disruptive effect on these routines and was likely to be interpreted by the boarders as punishment and resented accordingly:

> A group of us were working in the field. Suddenly a row blew up: Mark claimed that Olivia had been throwing clods of earth at him and he immediately began to retaliate. Robert (co-worker) intervened ... Robert told Mark that he expected Mark to show more maturity than to retaliate in response to Olivia's childishness. Mark eventually calmed down but then struck up a 'confidential' conversation with me which was spiced with threats to leave [Parkneuk]. Mark asked me where he could find a friend; by a 'friend' I took him to mean someone who would take his side and not be critical of him...

Gadamer (1976) has written of the disruptive effect of psychoanalytic interpretations in similar terms:

> The psychoanalyst leads the patient into the emancipatory reflection that gets behind the conscious superficial interpretations, breaks through the masked self-understanding, and sees through the repressive function of social taboos. But what happens when he uses the same kind of reflection in a situation in which he is not the doctor but a partner in a game? Then he will fall out of his social role! A game partner who is always 'seeing through' his game partner, who does not take seriously what they are standing for, is a spoil-sport whom one shuns.

Faswells and Ravenscroft

These two residential psychiatric units can be discussed together since they followed parallel approaches to therapy even though, as we saw in the last chapter, one of the communities was able to operationalise that approach much more successfully than the other at the time McKeganey conducted his fieldwork.

In general terms both communities can be seen to follow similar lines to Ashley and to the day hospital in that each community sought to hold up a mirror to the subject and to offer him or her the opportunity to experiment with different behaviour patterns and different forms of social relationships. We need not reiterate these similarities here; instead we will concentrate on those aspects of reality confrontation at Faswells and Ravenscroft which differentiate practice at those two communities from our earlier discussions of Ashley and the day hospital.

Redefinitions expressed at Faswells and Ravenscroft were more likely to contain psychoanalytic elements; the image of the resident reflected back in the reality confrontation was more likely to highlight unconscious or unacknowledged motives and feelings. For example, on one occasion a Ravenscroft small group leader had interpreted the feelings underlying the group as being unacknowledged anger at a staff member who was soon to leave the community. One of the residents who had felt a particularly close tie to the staff member replied by commenting that for her 'the community always felt different when Karen was on duty' and that her own 'feelings are not those of anger but at not wishing to say or do anything that would hurt her (i.e. Karen).' But the group leader commented: 'Well, I think there's a part of you that does want to and I think you're finding it tremendously difficult to acknowledge that that is how you feel.'

It was not that staff at Ashley or at the day hospital discounted the importance for treatment of the insight that residents and patients might gain from such psychoanalytic interpretations, nor that such interpretations were not voiced. The day hospital was catering for a wide range of patients including some, such as the elderly bereaved, with whom intensive group psychotherapy was not anticipated and whom it was felt could assimilate new behaviour patterns piecemeal without the necessity for developing insight into their previous pathogenic behaviour. As at Ashley, patient/resident insight was not devalued but was always tied, Gestalt-fashion, to personality and behaviour change.

A second difference in practice at Faswells and Ravenscroft, compared to our other communities practising reality confrontation, was the tendency not to orchestrate therapy by the instrumental use of reality confrontation. As in any group therapy setting, residents could feel the pressures of long group silences and it was certainly not staff practice to relieve the tensions that these silences could generate, but neither was it staff practice to orchestrate and focus pressure on particular individuals. There may be a tie-in (we are speculating) between this and our previous point: certainly, there is a strong non-directive tradition in psychoanalysis which stresses the responsibility of the therapists to *respond* to volitional patient behaviour. At Faswells reality confrontations offered in the large groups which might orchestrate further therapeutic work were often discouraged as disrupting the practical governmental function of the large groups. Thus the Faswells consultant commented to a colleague in the wake of one large group:

> I think we need to spend an evening discussing the role of interpretations in the large group meeting. When Dr Brown was here he suggested that there should be no interpretations offered in the big group. I didn't agree with that as it did not seem to me to correspond with reality. However, I do feel that interpretations need to be very limited. In today's meeting, as with last week, we had a situation where what was really a matter of practical decision-making was almost torpedoed by your flood of interpretations. A decision was reached on what was really a practical matter in spite of your intervention.

At Ravenscroft, although the expected length of resident stay (6 months) was only marginally longer than that at the day hospital or Ashley (4 months), there were relatively few attempts to orchestrate occasions of therapy. It was felt that day-to-day community activities like the cooking group would generate autonomously occasions for therapy to which staff could respond. We can take the conduct of the art therapy sessions as an example of the volitional approach to therapy at Ravenscroft.

In each art therapy session the therapist would suggest a single theme which each resident was expected to bear in mind; they were not expected to attempt a literal representation but to allow the theme to suggest images in their minds. Half an hour's painting was followed by one and a half hour's discussion, dealing with each work in turn. A portfolio of each resident's work was kept in the staff room as material for periodic art therapy reviews with individual residents and time was also made available in staff meetings for the therapist to present and discuss a selection of current work. There would be no attempt to anticipate a topic for therapy by suggesting different themes to different residents, the therapist would simply take what each resident had offered and draw out the implicit or unacknowledged messages to be found within each work.

Thus, on the theme of 'accidents', Graham drew an enlarged grey-shaded human egg surrounded by sperms. Graham, in discussion, remarked that 'the meaning of the picture was clear for everyone to see' – that his own birth had been an accident. The art therapist responded firstly by pointing out that the egg, although surrounded by sperm, had not been penetrated, and secondly that the colours used made the egg look cold and bleak, incapable of sustaining life. Graham agreed that leaving the egg unfertilised reflected his own sense of his life as somehow lacking a crucial ingredient, of being lifeless and incomplete.

Both Faswells and Ravenscroft followed a reality-confronting approach to therapy. Indeed the relative infrequency of planned interventions to orchestrate any therapeutic denouement places these two communities closer to the polar extremity along our axis of therapeutic approaches than any of our other candidate communities.

Conclusion

Beginning with an account of the recalcitrance of residents' social worlds to reality construction, we draw a distinction of emphasis in approaches to resocialisation. Some of our study communities (Ashley, the day hospital, Faswells and Ravenscroft) we have characterised as employing a reality-confronting approach. The other communities (Beeches, the concept house, Camphill and Parkneuk) we have characterised as instrumental communities. However, all these communities employed a mix of therapeutic approaches – our distinction is relative rather than absolute.

In conclusion we should attempt to clarify the conceptual basis of our distinction.

Ken Morrice has summarised as follows the process of reality construction through reality confrontation:

> As patients interact they reveal socially inept patterns of behaviour which are often characteristic of them, not only in the life of the therapeutic community, but also in terms of outside

> relationships with family and friends. Reality confrontation implies that the individual's conduct is reflected back to him in the hope that he will accept the interpretation and modify the offending behaviour. (Morrice, 1979, p. 55)

We might distinguish four sequentially-related aspects of this process: first there is the revelation of the resident's problem(s), as redefined by fellow community members; second, the bringing of this redefinition to the resident's attention; third, the acceptance by the resident of this redefinition; and fourth, a volitional change in resident behaviour.

Taking each of these aspects in turn, we can recall how various practices (such as the refusal of a supervisory staff role and the tolerance of consequent disruption) may ensure the re-enactment before practitioners' eyes of those pathogenic behaviour patterns that characterised the resident's life before his or her arrival at the community. The outside world is brought into the community and made visible for all to see; it is no longer part of the unremarked underlife of an institution or overlaid by the mechanical performance of hospital ward routines. The community is fashioned into a *speculum mundi*, a mirror of the world.

Likewise, bringing a redefinition to the resident's attention is not a matter of passively holding up a mirror to one absently or wilfully looking elsewhere, but rather involves directing that person's gaze as forcefully as is necessary. As we have shown, reality confrontation embraces many different presentational strategies from the gentle and ironical through to the vividly denunciatory. The staff-resident relationship remains under all circumstances a strategic power relationship and staff may choose from among various techniques of power the means to direct the resident's attention.

The bringing of a redefinition to the resident's attention is the core of reality confrontation, namely making the subject the observer of his or her own behaviour – the promotion of resident reflectivity. Again we follow Schutz in recognising that the greater part of human activity is routinised activity, where courses of action are not consciously deliberated but are unthinkingly followed as a matter of course, and where interpretations of situations are simple and unconsidered rather than a topic for scrutiny and investigation (Schutz, 1970). Then the mere interruption of this world of routine working, the questioning by others of what was formerly unproblematic and unconsidered, is in itself a possible stimulus for behavioural change. For example, the resident's previous interpretation of the situation may have been over-simple and vestigial precisely because it was unconsidered – it had only that degree of clarity and elaboration required by the resident's purpose at hand; by having the interpretation called into question the resident's purpose at hand is automatically changed and the interpretation may now be seen as inadequate and even erroneous. A search may then be embarked upon by the resident for a new or a more elaborate interpretation of the situation with a different associated course of action.

The view of resident behaviour that is being reflected back to the resident is no straightforward visual image but a particular and selective representation of the resident's behaviour. The resident, naturally enough, may incline to a different view. However, the likelihood of the resident's acceptance of a given redefinition may be increased in several ways. Thus, prior staff meetings may have established the redefinition as a joint and mutually agreed case-picture of the resident in question. Further, dissent from staff redefinitions may itself be redefined as further evidence of a resident's personality and relational problems – Sharp (1975) uses Berger and Luckmann's (1967) term 'nihilation' to describe this self-fulfilling aspect of staff redefinitional work.

Yet perhaps most influential in the promotion of resident acceptance of a redefinition is the role of the resident's peer group. As Schutz has shown (Schutz and Luckmann, 1974, pp. 59–92), following Cooley (1983), and Mead (1934), the subjects experience themselves through their associates and their associates experience themselves through the subject. It is not simply that subjects are aware of the expectations their associates have of them, but rather that subjects internalise and take over for their own the perceptions that their associates have of them. It is this assumption by subjects of the experience of themselves transmitted by others that Cooley has termed the 'looking glass self' – coming to see oneself as others see one. Thus when all a resident's associates, peer group as well as staff, draw attention to and describe a resident's conduct in similar terms, then it is more likely that the resident will come to see his or her own conduct through their eyes, than if only some of the resident's associates (the staff) were to engage in reality confrontation. The lack of a subcultural buttress to any alternative view of one's conduct strengthens the likelihood of resocialisation to the staff view.

To draw a redefinition to the resident's attention, and to promote the resident's acceptance of that redefinition, is to bring the resident to what we earlier described as the pivot of this therapeutic approach, namely volitional behaviour change. This situation of choice is not free of constraints – the right choice will be rewarded, the wrong choice may lead to further reality confrontation – but it is nevertheless an act of volition.

The promotion of reflectivity and emphasis on volitional behavioural change is in sharp contrast with the instrumental approach, where behavioural change is sought, one might almost say by stealth, certainly by the avoidance of reflection, lest the reflecting resident be moved to oppose the behaviour change being desired by the therapist. Staff sought behavioural change not through emphasising and enlarging the scope the resident has for volitional activity, but rather by restricting resident volition through subjecting what were previously areas of autonomous resident activity to scrutiny and control. The instrumental approach seeks to change resident behaviour by controlling the environment in which the behaviour occurs, by instructing the resident in new behaviour patterns, by rewarding the adoption of those behaviour patterns, and by monitoring and intervening in resident performance in order to ensure successful task completion. It is expected that these new behaviour patterns may then be inculcated by repetition and applied beyond the controlled environment of the community by 'graduating' residents.

In its essentials the instrumental approach aims at a reversal of the drive toward greater reflectivity that we described as a component of reality confrontation: the instrumental approach seeks to make these new behaviour patterns what Schutz called 'habitual possessions', routines that are unthinkingly followed under all typical circumstances. Residents are expected to react rather than reflect.

The adoption of a new social reality is no sudden transition; it proceeds through various recognisable stages. The discussion of these various treatment stages is the topic for our next chapter.

Chapter 4
Resident progress

Introduction

Assessments of the success of therapeutic intervention are sometimes treated in academic writing as if they were solely of concern to the research worker and the policy-maker, whereas of course such assessments are pre-eminently the concern of the client and the practitioner – the client for obvious reasons, and the practitioner for the scarcely less obvious reason that he or she must monitor the response to previous interventions in order to formulate an appropriate intervention for current or future circumstances. The actual content of everyday practice depends on continuing and continuous assessments of residents.

In popular imagery the success of therapeutic intervention is either a matter of precise measurement ('the temperature has fallen, nurse: the crisis has passed!') or so obvious that assessment is superfluous (the patient took up his bed and walked). In most areas of the therapeutic enterprise – and therapeutic communities are no exception – assessing the efficiency of different interventions is a more problematic affair, although, as we shall see, both measurement and obviousness play their part.

Staff assessments of residents in therapeutic communities are both recurrent and problematic. They may be set out in considerable detail, as in the formal 'resident reviews' found in some communities, or they may be a fleeting judgment made in the midst of the hurly-burly of community life. They are subject to contest; they tend to cumulate; they may be private but they are frequently shared and are often a collective construct.

Assessment cannot occur without some standard of comparison, implicit or explicit. Indeed, according to Schutz, all interpretation proceeds by reference to the individual's stock of knowledge, composed of a multitude of typifications (Schutz, 1962b). Assessments therefore embody notions of resident progress, notions of how residents should come ideally to respond and behave. In different communities progress will be visualised and recognised in different ways. In some communities an important component in the notion of progress is the increasing ability of residents to evidence their assimilation of the social world of the community by reproducing accounts of individual and collective behaviour which recognisably approach other accounts the resident has heard spoken by staff and senior residents. In other communities more attention in the assessment of progress is given to increasing resident competence in the performance of prescribed tasks and in set social situations.

This chapter compares the different conceptions of resident progress found in different communities. In effect, we shall compare how community members construct residents' 'success' or 'progress' in the course of everyday community activities – a research strategy advocated by Rawlings (1981). We begin with an examination of the different approaches employed in two communities (the day hospital and Parkneuk). The distinction we draw between communities in this chapter stems in turn from the distinction drawn in the previous chapter between reality-confronting and instrumental communities, and once more we shall find that we are not dealing with an absolute distinction but rather one of differential emphasis.

As we have already seen, communities vary considerably in the typical length, shape, and stages of residents' careers. Leaving aside unilateral decisions by residents to terminate their careers by hurried departure, contrasting conceptions of resident progress may partly determine intercommunity variations in career patterns. In the final section of the chapter we shall consider systematically this link between notions of resident progress and residents' career patterns.

Progress at the day hospital

Broadly speaking, the notions of patient progress operating in the day hospital entailed the patients' transition through two successive stages. The first stage was the patients' assimilation into the new social world of the community, with new background assumptions and new prescriptions for behaviour. The second stage was the patients' application of the new behaviour patterns learned in the day hospital to their old social world, their lives outside the day hospital. We shall examine each of these in turn.

Assimilation into a new social world implies more than a passive behavioural conformity. The latter is quickly achieved. We have already instanced how a patient on his first day in the day hospital was able to conduct himself quite adequately in the weekly encounter group whilst muttering 'What the hell's going on?'; studies of traditional psychiatric hospital regimes have repeatedly emphasised the ability of patients to adopt an outward passive behavioural conformity with the hospital regime whilst pursuing their own objectives and gratifications (see Goffman, 1968, pp. 157–266; Braginsky, Braginsky, and Ring, 1969).

Assimilation into a new social world entails a process of reality construction along the lines described in the previous chapter. Specifically, in the day hospital it involved getting the patient to orient to the doings of the community ('the group') as the 'paramount' or 'accent reality' (the terms are Schutz's, see Schutz, 1970), to disattend to previous preoccupations and to focus on the 'here and now' of events within the community. We can illustrate the argument by reference to three fieldnotes describing some of the contributions of one patient, Helen, over the course of a few days:

Note 1

Helen spoke about her worries about what was going on at home (were her two kids giving the newly engaged child-minder hell?). She apologised for speaking about home concerns, saying she had been pulled up for this before, but didn't know how to talk about what was going on in the group. This sounded like a request for guidance, though none was given. She also spoke about the silences and how she felt compelled to fill them. Simon (staff) replied that in responding in this way she deliberately set herself up for criticism. Helen asked Simon to explain. He replied 'No way' ... In the afternoon she returned to this topic ...

Note 2

(Following Eddie's description of his previous suicide attempt.) Helen asked Eddie how he was feeling now. This is a common technique to deflect patients from consideration of their problems in the past, or outside the group, towards groupwork ... It was interesting to see such a technique used by a patient ... who last week had bemoaned her failure to focus on the group rather than outside it.

Note 3

In the morning Helen spoke about her difficulty in getting off pills . . . She looked very care-worn and weepy. Said she felt the group was giving her something and she wouldn't have made the effort to give up the pills on her own. Tina (patient) shared, saying she was trying to give up alcohol . . . In the afternoon Tim (patient) was trying to console Mike (patient) who was saying he felt lonely now his seniors (as patients) had left. Tim said he would feel lonely when Mike left. Helen picked on this, saying Tim could surely get closer to her and her fellow, less senior, patients. The discussion drifted away but someone . . . brought it back by telling Helen she thought she'd sounded quite angry. Helen agreed, saying that she usually bottled up her anger, afraid of provoking an angry response and a scene: she would turn her anger in on herself but eventually it would find an outlet, she would blow her top and feel wretched. Edith (staff) helped her by quoting Len (staff) to the effect that when anger's inside you it feels like a lion but it generally comes out like a mouse.

I asked her how she felt now: she said she felt a lot better – it was the first time she's been angry in the group and accepted that she was angry (she referred to last week when Oliver (staff) had said that Helen was angry with him and Helen had denied it, but now realised that she was); Tim had accepted her anger and not thrown it back at her – she felt that she could now let out her anger as it occurred instead of turning it in and storing it up. She asked if this made sense: we said it did . . . Helen remarked that it seemed silly to feel angry with Tim, but she did . . .

We can draw several points out of these notes on Helen's contributions. Firstly, and most importantly, there is the shift, in the space of only a few days, in Helen's apparent preoccupation with her family to 'the group'. The group is no longer an artificial entity, an heterogeneous collection of comparative strangers, but is now an important reference group (without whom Helen would not have struggled to give up her pills) capable of eliciting strong emotional reactions from her. It seemed silly to feel angry with Tim, but she did. Bloor, in his turn, came to recognise, with some surprise, how strongly attached he felt to his fellow group members in the course of his fieldwork.

To be specific about this shift in Helen's attentions, it is not that Helen has leapt from one finite province of reality to another. Rather she lives in several provinces of reality simultaneously but at any one time only one is paramount. Provinces of reality that were formerly paramount recede to the horizon and a new theme becomes paramount, although that which is now horizontal in the field of consciousness remains open to recall to a paramount position (Schutz, 1970, pp. 1–12).

A second point to be derived from the notes on Helen concerns the fact that there are particular conversational devices in use in the day hospital to promote this Gestalt emphasis on the 'here and now'. One such device, used twice in the above extracts, was to ask 'how do you feel now?' (emphasis on the 'now'). Another device was to offer some personal judgment (perhaps critical, perhaps approbatory) and follow it with the question 'how do you feel about that?' So widespread were these conversational devices that patients came to adopt them as a matter of course. One patient laughed about how she had unwittingly given pause to her acquaintances outside the day hospital by peppering her conversation with the question 'how do you feel about that?'.

Like all institutions, the day hospital had its own argot and linguistic conventions. Terms like 'working', 'stuck', and 'sharing' had situated meanings (for an extended analysis of the ways in which the term 'sharing' was used in the day hospital, see Wootton, 1977). Competent performance in the group depended on grasping the situated meanings of these terms, phrases, questions, and conventions and using them in turn. The situated meanings could not be exhaustively specified since, as in all terms, there was a degree of residual indeterminacy. However, competent usage was a badge of group membership, which new patients took time to acquire.

The reason why competent usage of day hospital argot may be seen as a mark of patient progress lies in the fact that language is constitutive of social reality: repeated references to current feeling-states constitute those feeling-states as a central topic of concern, the paramount reality. This leads us to the third point we can draw from the fieldnotes on Helen's contributions, namely her increasing reflectivity on her feelings and behaviour ('Helen agreed, saying she usually bottled up her anger ...', and so on). As we saw in the previous chapter, a crucial component of the treatment process in reality-confronting communities is the promotion of reflectivity and of the possibility of adopting new and less pathogenic patterns of behaviour.

Our final point concerns Helen's reappraisal of her previous contributions ('last week when Oliver had said that Helen was angry with him Helen had denied it, but now realised that she was'). Similar remarks could be heard on occasion from many other patients – that they only now realised what the purpose of the groups was, that everything they'd said in the groups initially was, they now realised, a load of rubbish, and so on. The newly arrived patient encounters frequent 'reality disjunctures' (Pollner, 1975), views of the world which contrast sharply with the patient's own. As resocialisation proceeds the patient embraces those previously disjunctive perceptions and may well take the further step of disavowing previously expressed views: the patient now sees that the disjunctive view was really the correct one all along. Berger and Kellner (1970) have analysed in similar terms the joint resocialisation of marriage partners and the disavowal of pre-marital viewpoints.

The first stage of patient progress in the day hospital was the assimilation of the patient into the new social world of the community and this assimilation can be seen to have several components: orienting to the 'here and now' of the group as the paramount reality, competence in the reality-constituting argot of the community, reflection upon one's previously unthinkingly assumed behaviour patterns, and disavowal of one's earlier perceptions.

Before proceeding to a discussion of the second stage of patient progress, however, we should sound a note of caution. All assessments of patient progress are provisional and defeasible: patients may display all the marks of progress shown by Helen above and yet still be judged 'stuck', in that staff may see in the patient's behaviour further evidence which overturns a favourable interpretation of patient progress. The likeliest way for such an overturning to occur is where the patients are seen as having assimilated into the community but are thought to exercise a subversive and antagonistic or manipulative influence on the groups. For example, at one point during Bloor's fieldwork, in order to avoid overloading the groups during a period when the numbers of patients in the day hospital had diminished, the initial Monday morning group would begin with a discussion as to which of those staff members available would be selected to take part in the groups that week. In one Monday morning group the following exchanges occurred in respect of Tim's preferences for certain staff members:

> Oliver (staff) turned to Tim (patient) and said he was surprised that he hadn't stated his preferences as regards staff members because he'd been complaining last week about decisions being imposed by the staff. Tim then said he wanted Len in the group and he didn't want Oliver and Edith. Both his want for Len and his wish to be rid of Oliver and Edith were subsequently used as material for discussion . . . in wanting to swop father-figure Len for father-figure Oliver, he was being destructive; since he knew Len couldn't work in the groups (at that time), his stated preference was an attempt to wound Oliver and Edith just to provoke a response. At lunchtime (when no staff were present) Tim got a laugh from his fellow patients by saying that next week staff should be forced to say which patients they wanted to work with and patients should say whether they would be available or not.

Relatedly, a judgment of patient progress may be overturned where it is thought that a patient has assimilated to the community but that he or she is taking an excessive interest in other patients' difficulties. When staff in therapeutic communities use the term 'patient therapist' they do so, on occasion at least, with critical connotations: such patients may be thought to be hiding behind others' difficulties or else to be using patients with similar problems as an indirect and unsatisfactory means of exploring their own difficulties.

The second stage of resident progress contrasts sharply with the first stage in comprising a refocusing on the patient's relationships outside the day hospital and the application of lessons learned in the group to those outside relationships. Consider the remarks of Stephanie, a senior patient suffering a bereavement, and the staff's approbatory response:

> She now felt that she finally accepted her husband's death – he wasn't coming back. She spoke sensibly about the things that she had brought from her own home to her mother's which had upset her, like the double bed – she was going to sell it now and buy a single. Her Mum had kept the baby till Sunday evening and she'd been surprised how she'd really felt lost without him on Sunday –

> she accepted him now . . . She'd said previously that she felt attracted to Oliver (staff) because he was so like her husband, but now she felt attracted to him independently of his resemblance to her husband. Kim (medical student on placement) asked about her feelings about meeting other men and was this one reason why she felt unhappy about going out – frightened lest she meet a replacement? She hadn't thought of it that way, but it might be so she thought. When this was recapitulated in the staff group, Len was very pleased – definite progress he thought.

Drawing on this and similar expressions of staff approval of patient conduct, we can suggest two grounds for staff seeing 'definite progress' in Stephanie's case. In the first place we can note Stephanie's readiness to *act* to change her life circumstances ('selling the double bed'). Enhanced patient understanding of his or her situation was not greatly valued by staff unless it was accompanied by patient action to change unrealistic expectations and pathogenic relationships. Relatedly, we can note Stephanie's readiness to learn the lesson of the immediate social world of the group (that she is attracted to Oliver for his own qualities, not for a fancied resemblance to her dead husband) and preparedness to apply that lesson to the social world she will inhabit outside the day hospital (she will meet other men to whom she is attracted). To so apply the new-learned perspectives and prescriptions of the therapeutic community to life outside the community often entails the renunciation of previously held viewpoints that are now seen as 'unrealistic', as with Stephanie's previous unwillingness to come to terms with her husband's death.

Taken together, the first and second stages of patient progress constitute a complex double switch. The patient is first of all weaned away from his or her old world to the new world of the group, portrayed as a world of warm and caring relationships qualitatively different from the world that the patient has left behind. But then the patient comes to see that this new world has many parallels with the old world and that the understandings that have been achieved in the day hospital may also illuminate the patient's situation outside the day hospital, and the behaviour patterns experimented with in the group may also be applied outside the group.

Elsewhere, Bloor and Fonkert (1982) have described as a process of 'reality exploration' the gradual realisation by patients of the parallels between the community and their previous social world.

Patients in the day hospital and residents in Fonkert's concept house exploring the prescriptions for patient and resident behaviour found these prescriptions to be incipiently contradictory, to be provisional and defeasible: there were limits to permissiveness, limits to care and concern, and limits to democracy. Angry accusations from patients and residents that staff were behaving inconsistently were likely to meet the response that staff accepted that they sometimes acted inconsistently and sometimes failed to live up to the expectations placed upon them. Staff would stress that their behaviour only mirrored that found in everyday social life and that patients must learn to come to terms with inconsistency in others: the therapeutic community offered them an opportunity to learn to react to such disappointments in a less pathogenic manner.

Notions of resident progress in the day hospital therefore involved two stages – firstly, the successful assimilation of the patient into the culture of the community (a process of reality construction), and secondly, the application of the lessons learned in the community to the patient's social world outside (a process of reality exploration).

Progress at Parkneuk

Co-workers' notions of boarders' progress at Parkneuk were in sharp contrast to those at the day hospital – here there was no two-stage process. Since only a minority of Parkneuk boarders were expected to return to life on the 'outside' rather than graduate to an adult community such as Newton Dee village, there was less necessity for Parkneuk co-workers to concern themselves with the rehabilitative issue that loomed so large at the day hospital: that of getting the patients to apply the lessons learned in the therapeutic community to their relationships outside the day hospital. Similarly, since the Parkneuk boarders were normally expected to stay in the community for several years (rather than the four months of the day hospital patients), their assimilation was a less pressing concern.

The co-workers at Parkneuk believed that it was possible for themselves and the boarders to create a social environment that was superior to that available outside the community ('At [Parkneuk] we ought to be able to make a better way of living, a better way of life than life on the outside ... we shouldn't just be trying to make a creative satisfying life for the residents, but for the co-workers as well'). This Utopian vision, reinforced by the absence in most cases of a need to rehabilitate boarders, allowed the Parkneuk co-workers to be critical of other therapeutic approaches:

> Robert (co-worker) . . . talks about one of their new boarders who has apparently had a very difficult relationship with her parents. Her social worker has been encouraging her to focus on her relationship with her parents, believing that once she has worked this out then she will be able to go forward. At Parkneuk, on the other hand, their focus has been on getting her to create new social relationships, to submerge the past in the present. Robert said that eventually he had to speak to the social worker about it because they were pulling in different directions . . .

Since the past is to be submerged and the future for the boarder is seen as 'a better way of living' at Parkneuk and similar communities, resident progress can be judged solely on the basis of increased proficiency, sociability and autonomy in the domestic life of the therapeutic community. The following fieldnotes document judgments on the progress over time of Kenny, a Down's Syndrome adolescent:

> <u>Note 1 (21.3.77 – pilot study)</u>
>
> Talking with Robert and a visitor from another community. Kenny goes past wheeling a barrow. Robert remarks on how much he has advanced since he first arrived [at Parkneuk], when a task like wheeling a barrow was something he was quite unable to manage. Remarks about Kenny's progress have been made several times in my hearing before: e.g., Nina has spoken of his initial utter uncooperativeness . . . However, Kenny still seems pitifully ill-equipped for the world: it only makes sense to talk of his progress in terms of his continuing in some sheltered environment.
>
> This morning Kenny went to the bathroom to clean his teeth. To wet his toothbrush he decided to turn both taps full on. He then decided to go to the toilet. Nicky found him sitting on the toilet, feet in the air, toothbrush in his mouth, surrounded by water.
>
> <u>Note 2: (undated)</u>
>
> Tom says Kenny brings a lot of happiness to the house: 'if you're

feeling a bit fed up you can always go and have a talk to Kenny.' They think he is much improved – coming down to breakfast and finding his place not set and no breakfast ready, he immediately began getting it himself. Tom spoke of an impromptu entertainment staged by Kenny and Robert the other day, based on the very sinister way Kenny says 'cream crackers'.

Note 3: (20.2.78)

During the wiping up, Kenny will pick up a plate and a tea towel but then he will lean against the stove, chuckling to himself, and continually wipe the same plate for ages until the wiping up is finished (by the others).

Note 4: (13.4.78)

While I was washing up Kenny picked up a ladle to wipe dry but silently handed it back to me when he saw I hadn't washed all the food off it.

Note 5: (20.1.79 – return visit)

Progress. Kenny is now working in the weavery. He has mastered the sequence of activities although he is painfully slow.

These fieldnote extracts illustrate three related components in assessments of Kenny. Firstly, there were judgments of competence in task-performance, be it wheeling a barrow or weaving cloth. This included rationality in task performance – merely ritualistic repetition was devalued. Secondly, there were judgments of autonomy in task performance – getting one's own breakfast unbidden. And finally, there were judgments about the boarder's sociability and social relations within the Parkneuk foster family.

The marks of boarders' progress were not universal criteria, but rather were peculiar to individual boarders. For example, co-workers would expect more rapid progress from disturbed boarders than from a Down's Syndrome boarder like Kenny. Some marks of progress were laid down, programme-like, for boarders to aim at (like Kenny's weaving), while others simply involved the recognition of progress in the boarders' response to some serendipitous event (the non-appearance of Kenny's breakfast). In both cases, of course, co-workers must redefine some mundane event or activity as having a potential for therapy. At Parkneuk such redefinitions, whether they were the planning of boarders' activities or the recognition of a successful initiative, were typically abbreviated and highly glossed, with implicit appeals to the 'obviousness' of the redefinition and the superfluity of elaboration. On Victor's attending motor cycling proficiency classes, Robert simply remarked in one of the (rare) co-workers' meetings, 'it would really be good if he passed his test. Think what it would do for him.'

This is not to say that the progress of boarders was indeed 'obvious'. We are reporting here on appeals, statements which attract support because of their level of generality and their invitation to the hearer to fill out the sense of the speaker's statement (Garfinkel, 1967). Particular knowledge and particular skills are required to perceive and to programme these marks of progress. Particular knowledge of Kenny's capabilities in wiping up was required to invest with significance Kenny's return of a dirty ladle. Also, the programming of boarders' activities would require the skill to break down a task into component parts which might challenge a boarder's capabilities. So, for example, it might be beyond either of two boarders to sow a row of carrot seed, but one boarder might be capable of going first to hoe the shallow drill and another of going third to fill in the drill, if the co-worker went second to thin-sow the seed.

We have remarked previously that in its essentials the therapeutic approach at Parkneuk was one of creating benign routines within a foster family environment. It was a learned skill of co-workers to see within these routines the possibility of enhancing boarders' capabilities and monitoring these same routines for marks of progress. Assessment of boarders' progress was purely in terms of their performance within these routines.

The lack of any external yardstick of performance was recognised by the co-workers to be a problem, particularly in their dealings with referral agencies:

> Nicky said she and Robert had to write a report on Victor recently and she had found it very difficult. She finds it impossible to say how far his apparent improvement is simply a successful adjustment to life at Parkneuk community and would be immediately lost if he shifted elsewhere.

In respect of that minority of boarders judged potentially capable of independence outside Parkneuk, the co-workers recognised that such boarders faced problems of transition and endeavoured, where possible, to make special arrangements to ease these.

The contrasts that are evident between notions of progress current at Parkneuk and those employed in the day hospital are clearly associated with the different treatment approaches that were set out in the previous chapter. Recall Robert's difference of opinion with the new boarder's social worker. Likewise, it is only in a reality-confronting community, such as the day hospital, that one mark of progress is the reflection of the patient on his or her previously unthinkingly adopted patterns of behaviour, since a central aim of treatment in such communities is to make the resident the observer of his or her own behaviour.

However, a further source of contrasts between Parkneuk and the day hospital may lie in the rejection by the former of any substantial rehabilitative role. Rehabilitation poses particularly acute problems for resocialising institutions such as therapeutic communities (as Rapoport recognised in his research at the Henderson Hospital thirty years ago, Rapport, 1960): no sooner has the resident been converted to a new world of caring social relationships than he or she must be prepared to return to the now devalued old world from whence he or she came. Communities such as the day hospital which accept a large rehabilitative function must operate with a two-stage concept of resident progress if they are to overcome this tension.

Progress in other communities

Having examined in some detail contrasting conceptions of resident progress in two communities, we can depict notions of resident progress in the other study communities more briefly, concentrating on those aspects which diverge from our findings relating to the Day Hospital and Parkneuk. We will look firstly at the remaining instrumental communities – Beeches, the concept house, and the Camphill community.

At Beeches, as at Parkneuk, resident improvement was judged by behavioural indicators – task performance, autonomy of performance, and social relations. Similarly, these judgments were frequently heavily glossed, self-evident to all competent staff members. Consider this fieldnote on the performance of a very withdrawn resident at a disco during the annual house holiday:

> When we arrived I found Ianthe (resident) dancing away at the disco with a very happy smile on her face: I signalled my amazement to staff members who nodded and smiled. She danced continuously for the next three hours . . . At various points during the evening staff members would briefly comment, 'Look at Ianthe, isn't she great?' 'She's still going, look. See how happy she looks?' It was seen as self-evident that Ianthe's enjoyment of this social occasion was a sign of progress. . .

These fleeting judgments might be much amplified (and even disputed) during the resident review section of the weekly staff meeting when two residents would be discussed in detail each week. However, these resident reviews were naturally more concerned with current problems in residents' performance (and how to rectify them) than with resident progress as such.

Judgments of improvements in resident task performances were facilitated by the extensive specification and standardisation of residents' tasks – for example, by the written lists of cleaning jobs in each of the public rooms, and by the very detailed recipes that each resident had to follow repetitively on his or her turn on the meal rota. Precise measurement of performance (and therefore improvement) was most closely approached in the psycho-education-influenced ceramics class and in the formal education sessions, the latter conducted by a trained teacher.

Where practice at Beeches differed most significantly from that at Parkneuk was in the way judgments of resident progress were tied to promotion in the house hierarchy. Since each promotion led to increasing resident autonomy (work experience outside the house, later bedtimes, own room) formal recognition of resident progress was thought to move the resident automatically towards eventual rehabilitation by the progressive relinquishment of staff controls. Although Beeches staff shared the concern of the day hospital staff with rehabilitation, there was no necessity for a two-stage notion of resident progress since the progressive rehabilitation of the resident was thought to be an automatic consequence of rewarding improved task performance.

In the Camphill community there was something of a dual system of child assessment. Whilst the co-workers in the houses would make on-going judgments of children's progress in similar terms to those of the co-workers in Parkneuk, the formal responsibility for assessing the child lay with senior members of the community – the child's house parent (the senior co-worker in the house), the school teachers, those responsible for administering the various specialist therapies, and, pre-eminently, the doctors manning the community clinics where the child would be seen at regular intervals. Assessment at the clinics was a matter of clinical judgment and proceeded on lines that were similar in form to those found in any paediatric clinic. At least once a term every child would be seen by the medical consultant in the presence of the house parent and the dormitory parent; there would be written reports from the house and the school. The child would receive a physical examination and be examined on his or her performance of tests of motor function and the like. The medical consultant would then proceed to make any necessary changes in medication, recommend specific therapies, such as coloured light therapy, and suggest particular activities and exercises for the child to do within the house.

Formal judgments of the progress of the Camphill child were made by the medical consultant based on physical and behavioural indicators and reports of the child's social behaviour, and were derived from a corpus of knowledge that drew on both allopathic medicine and anthroposophy. We have already provided some materials on the anthroposophical elements in this corpus in Chapter 2 (see also McKeganey, 1984). An example of clinical judgments is provided below:

> The clinic takes place in the coffee room. Present are the house parent, medical consultant, senior co-worker, and the teacher and dormitory parent of the child being discussed. The house parent begins: 'She has no morality, she pinches food, goes through the adults' rooms and pinches alarm clocks. Both our budgerigars have been killed – we have no proof but we're fairly sure it was her. She has taken out one of the younger children and dumped him in the bushes. When you confront her she does not feel sorry.' The doctor listens intently to all this and then asks the school teacher how the child has been – 'There has been some improvement, one feels she wants to be here. At first I gave her lots of attention which she liked. She has difficulty concentrating, though, and in listening to what is being said.' Doctor, 'But she is not uncooperative.' Teacher, 'No, not now, but she was.'
>
> The doctor then asks for the child to be shown in. He chats to her and holds her hands as he does so. Afterwards the child is shown out. Doctor: 'Very interesting, her hands were cold and

wet. All over she gives the impression of being dirty, through and through. She has a very low self image which is in part of course psychological, but also physiological. Did you notice her hunched posture? I think it would be important to involve her in plays. It could be that she has had meningitis. Her ego has difficulty incarnating, which is perhaps why she is all over the place, since it is the ego which unites us. I would suggest using the Silica because she is so dark. D20 at noon and Argentum in the morning and evening and repeat that next term. Tell Katarin (Curative Eurythmist) to add the double D in her eurythmy and involve her in the drama groups. Right, so who's next?'

Such assessments form an important component (together with the availability of suitable placements) in deciding the eventual placement of the children when schooling finishes. Once again, parallel informal assessments are made by the co-workers living alongside the children, so that, for example, those children nearing school-leaving age and judged capable of living outside a mental subnormality hospital may be informally reintroduced to aspects of life outside the community by accompanying co-workers on house shopping expeditions and the like.

The concept house is again in something of a unique position. In the previous chapter we described the concept house as using reality confrontation techniques in the service of an instrumental approach to therapy. In considering assessments of resident progress we find the concept house to be something of a hybrid. Judgments of resident progress were based both on assimilation into the culture of the community (as in the day hospital) and on the completion of satisfactory standards of task performance (as at Parkneuk and Beeches). Assimilation would be judged on the extent to which fellow community members became an important reference group to the new resident, on competence in the argot of the community, on the ability to monitor and relate one's feelings, and on reappraisal of one's previous junkie existence. And task performance would be judged in respect of the very high standards demanded and overseen in the various work groups or departments. Failures in assimilation or tasks would be met by exhortations ('pull-ups'), denunciations ('haircuts'), demotion in the status hierarchy, and 'therapeutic measures' like sign-wearing. Satisfactory progress was rewarded correspondingly.

Nevertheless, judgments of resident progress in the concept house remained problematic. Because of the emphasis on social and behavioural conformity, and because of the high levels of supervision, all residents became agents of the normative system in the house, regardless of whether or not they endorsed it internally (see Sugarman, 1975). As a consequence, deviant residents would normally believe themselves to be completely isolated in their resistance, so that overt resistance to authority was very rare (outside the licence of the encounter groups) and could take very few forms other than premature departure, open or secret. Under such circumstances normal evidence of assimilation and conformity automatically becomes suspect – all progress can be feigned. Indeed, it is generally recognised that, despite the pull-ups, haircuts, seminars, and so on, new residents in concept houses only belatedly realise the immense changes expected of them.

Given this paradoxical possibility of feigned conformity within the pressure cooker of the concept house staff were likely to place particular emphasis on certain cues in making judgments about resident progress, the cues being idiosyncratic to particular residents and reflecting their particular problems as conceptualised by the staff. It was judged to be a mark of progress, for example, when a shy, withdrawn resident was heard shouting at her fellows. Among senior residents idiosyncratic cues denoting progress were comparatively unimportant, in these cases the important cues to which staff would attend were those indicating backsliding.

In contrast to the situation at Beeches, the concept house did not envisage progress towards rehabilitation as an automatic consequence of promotion in the status hierarchy. The house structure merely represented heterogeneous opportunities for calling forth desired qualities from different residents and so senior residents were as likely to be found working as crew members in the kitchens as they were to be occupying senior positions in the structure. In one sense, rehabilitation was not a concern in the concept house; this was a matter for the halfway house to which concept house residents would graduate. In another sense, the possibility of rehabilitation was constantly before residents since most of the staff were graduates from their own or other concept houses – every resident carries a field-marshall's baton in his knapsack.

We turn now to the remaining reality-confronting communities: Ashley, Ravenscroft and Faswells.

Staff at Ashley could be heard using a number of yardsticks of residents' progress which, taken together, amount to four sequential stages of progress. These four stages were, in staff terminology: 'settling in', 'talking in groups', 'using the house' and 'getting ready to leave'. Each term of course connotes and glosses a wide range of resident behaviour.

'Settling in' refers both to the new resident's familiarity with the routines of the house (the timetable and conduct of the work groups, the coffee groups, the weekly community meeting, and so on) and to the resident's assimilation into the peer group of his or her fellow residents. 'Settling in' therefore incorporates judgments of task performance (as in the instrumental communities) and judgments about the new resident's acceptance of fellow community members as an important reference group (as in Helen's behaviour at the day hospital).

The next stage of resident progress was 'talking in the groups', referring to the daily coffee groups and the weekly community meeting. Of course, not all resident talk was seen as equally valuable. The most valued contributions from relatively new residents were expressions of feelings ('something to work on', as the warden termed it), responses to the comments of others on the subject's behaviour (responses to reality confrontation), and descriptions or reflections by the subject on his or her own feelings and behaviour. Contributions of the latter type might only occur some weeks after the initial venting of anger and belligerent replies to reality confrontation. However, such reflectivity (paralleling marks of progress at the day hospital) often occurred as a direct consequence of immediately prior angry exchanges at Ashley.

That reflectivity could occur hard on the heels of the expression of feelings owed much to a particular feature of the Ashley programme – 'aftergroup'. Following the end of the weekly community meeting residents and staff alike would adjourn to the kitchen and sit around the table with mugs of tea to talk about how they personally had felt during the community meeting. The atmosphere was relaxed and informal with jokes and humorous recapitulations of incidents and events; indeed the aftergroup was partly designed to defuse the tensions of the community meeting. But the aftergroup was also designed to allow residents, within the relaxed atmosphere of a natural break, to describe for others what they had just been feeling. In the staff group that followed the aftergroup it was commonplace for staff to pass remarks such as that it was 'good' that some resident or other had felt able to say that they had been feeling really angry.

'Using the house' is a term that we have already met with and discussed in the description of therapeutic work at Ashley in the previous chapter. It refers to resident experimentation with new patterns of behaviour in the permissive environment of the house. Again there are parallels with the notions of patient progress operative in the day hospital.

Two quite different kinds of resident behaviour might be referred to by staff at Ashley as indicating that a resident was 'getting ready for leaving'. On the one hand, staff used the term in respect of moves by residents actually to prepare themselves for departure from the house (for example, looking for work or for accommodation), particularly where these moves were thought to be an application of lessons learned in the house (for example, in no longer expecting parents or other authority figures to organise one's life). On the other hand, staff might also use the term to redefine complaints or dissatisfaction from senior residents with aspects of the house regime. A senior resident who said he now felt bored with the community meetings was told that this was probably because he was no longer deriving much benefit from them, a sign that he was 'getting ready to leave'. Such staff remarks could, of course, be heard as a mechanism of social control, as the nihilation of dissent (see Chapter 5), but they could also be tied to the staff belief that residents could stay too long in the community, eventually ceasing to make further progress and 'messing up'. Comparable redefinitions of dissatisfaction from senior patients as indicative of progress could also be heard on occasion in the day hospital.

The first stage of patient progress found at the day hospital was also found at our two residential psychiatric units, Ravenscroft and Faswells: namely, the constitution of the community as an important reference group, the enhanced reflectivity respecting the subjects' feeling states and behaviour patterns, and the disavowal of earlier perceptions. However, at Ravenscroft and Faswells staff would also look for prior signs of resident progress: they believed that before residents could arrive at the 'reality construction' stage we documented earlier they must first recognise that they indeed had problems, particularly difficulties in their relationships with others, and that they must have some motivation to change these.

For residents to recognise that they had problems and be motivated to tackle them might be thought to be a pre-condition of therapy and in some communities (the day hospital included) this was a matter to be settled prior to the resident's admission, normally through the device of verbal 'contract', with the resident admitting in the course of the interview that he or she did indeed have problems and that he or she was committed to working on them. Such contracts were of course unenforceable and staff were clear that patients' initial conceptions of their problems would be sketchy and perhaps largely erroneous. They were also clear that patients' motivations to enter therapy would rarely be strong enough to sustain them throughout therapy without additional reinforcement in the course of treatment.

Only in specific and unusual circumstances would the day hospital staff accept patients in the absence of such recognition and commitment – an adolescent patient could constitute such an exception, for example. Staff at Ravenscroft and Faswells endorsed the desirability of establishing such contracts at admission, but in the case of Faswells, believed themselves so poorly served by referral agencies that they had to relax their admission criteria in order to maintain community numbers at a minimum level of viability. Under these circumstances many of the incoming residents could only be expected to recognise that they had problems and to develop the motivation to change their relations with others *in the course of treatment*. For residents to exhibit signs of such recognition and motivation therefore became a mark of progress. The possible signs of such initial progress were several and somewhat situation-specific. An alcoholic, for example, might concede that the reasons for his or her drinking behaviour lay in more than a mere physiological addiction. Or a patient with psychosomatic complaints might accept that he or she had more than just physical ailments.

Following these early judgments of resident progress, residents at Faswells and Ravenscroft would subsequently be assessed in similar terms to those described as the first stage of resident progress at the day hospital. However, the situation in respect of the second stage of progress at the day hospital – the application of lessons learned in the community to the residents' social situations outside the hospital – was rather less clear cut. Certainly there was ample evidence of such a stage at Ravenscroft, though at Faswells the situation was hampered by the lack of consensual staff judgments as to residents' progress towards rehabilitation. While Faswells staff could on occasion be heard questioning residents about their application of lessons learned within the community to their life outside the unit, there was a good deal of disagreement between staff as to which of the residents this ought realistically to be expected of. Indeed Faswells staff could repeatedly be heard lamenting the loss of agreed criteria for assessing residents' progress – a situation which they accepted had led to many residents remaining in the community long after they had learned to derive any benefit from participation in the life of the community. One of the nurses commented:

> Basically you can analyse and interpret all you like but now there's nothing left to work with. It's always the same old spiel. Time and again the same old stuff. We desperately need new people, you can see that. The time for talking is long gone now, there's only one thing left – action – and that, for most of them, is moving out.

The possible reasons why such residents were not moving out are discussed in Chapter 6. Here we can only note the absence of consensual staff judgments on the progress residents were making towards rehabilitation, and the obvious implications this held for the shaping of residents' careers in the community.

Variations in career patterns

Our object in this study has been to compare and contrast communities in terms of differences in their approaches to therapeutic work. An alternative comparative method would be that of examining differences between communities in typical patterns of resident careers, a strategy first suggested by Goffman (1968, p. 119), who used the term 'careers' to characterise the temporal progression of residents through institutions. Yet these two – therapeutic work and careers – are not independent: as the previous discussion has already implied, residents' career patterens in any one community will be influenced partly by the approach to therapeutic work adopted in that community; the medium for this influence will be the conceptions of resident progress associated with a given approach to therapeutic work. In the remainder of this chapter we shall aim to provide a conclusion to our previous discussion of different communities' conceptions of resident progress by examining the relationship between, on the one hand, approaches to therapeutic work and conceptions of resident progress, and, on the other hand, residents' career patterns.

However, before considering this relationship, it would be wise to consider a fourth factor, namely, the nature of the resident's difficulties and the influence these may have on approaches to therapeutic work, on conceptions of resident progress and on residents' career patterns.

There is a good case for ascribing a determining influence to the nature of the resident's difficulties. Clearly Kenny, the Down's syndrome adolescent at Parkneuk, would not have been a suitable candidate for the day hospital treatment approach. Kenny's problem (that of limited domestic, working and social skills) was a type of difficulty that the day hospital was less orientated towards treating. The treatment methods of the day hospital demanded minimum levels of perceptual ability that were probably beyond Kenny's capacities. Moreover, Kenny's rate of improvement was likely to be slow and so a lengthy resident career was inevitable.

Yet there is also a contrary case to be made. It might be argued with equal force that the treatment approach determines the nature of a resident's problems. These problems are not wholly self-evident: they are constructed by a process of redefinition such as we described in Chapter 3. Moreover, there is empirical evidence as well as theoretical argument. Ashley and Beeches were communities with contrasting treatment approaches but catered for an overlapping clientele. Whilst educationally subnormal adolescents were a majority at Beeches and a minority at Ashley, residents in both houses showed a considerable spread of intellectual abilities and attainments – similar problems were treated by contrasting methods.

There are certain conditions (for example, paranoia) which are widely agreed to be disqualified from any therapeutic community approach, but excluding such groups we would argue that the resident's condition is only a crucial determinant of the choice of treatment, or of the resident's career, at the extremes of the ability range and in respect of a very limited number of presenting problems. While elective mute-ism, for example, is not a condition suitable for a reality confrontation approach, Maxwell Jones (1982) nevertheless claims to have conducted a successful programme of therapeutic community work with psychogeriatric patients.

We shall turn now to the influence that the approach to therapeutic work, mediated through notions of resident progress, exerts on patterns of resident careers. The most notable aspect of residents' careers in any community is, of course, their typical length, and we can at once see that the typical length of residents' careers differs systematically between our two types of community – instrumental and reality-confronting. Taking the instrumental communities first, all of them are characterised by relatively extensive resident careers, while among the reality-confronting communities only the residents at Faswells had typical careers of comparable length.

This leads us to question the belief sometimes voiced in instrumental communities that the resocialisation of residents is necessarily a long-term project. Instead, it can be seen that resocialisation is only a long-term project if it is to be accomplished by certain methods (we leave aside the question of whether these methods are surer of success than others applicable within a shorter span of time). It must be a matter for speculation as to why the pursuit of an instrumental approach to therapy should be associated with relatively extended resident careers. Since the length of any one career will depend on staff judgments of resident progress, it seems possible that notions of progress centring on fine and progressive improvements in task performance may be responsible. Certainly, where these judgments are tied to progressive promotion in a resident status hierarchy (as they were at Beeches and the concept house) it seems almost axiomatic that residents' careers will also be lengthy in order to allow the time for residents to occupy and vacate each of these statuses.

A similar case can be made for Camphill, where, although there was not the same elaborate status hierarchy as in Beeches and the concept house, nevertheless the children were differentiated in the house and in school in terms of their ages. Progression through the Waldorf curriculum in the school, and from the junior to the senior dormitories in the house, would take place over a number of years rather than months.

Our remaining instrumental community (Parkneuk) eschewed a status hierarchy for residents and this might seem to strengthen the case that it is a reliance on marks of behavioural performance itself that produces lengthy resident careers. In Goffman's terminology each mark of resident progress becomes a 'career stage', and the more the career stages then, other things being equal, the longer the career. However, the case must remain 'not proven' since Parkneuk and Camphill community had only limited orientations toward rehabilitation – a state of affairs that also tends to lengthen residents' careers, as we have already seen in respect of Faswells.

It might be thought that patterns of defaulting – the premature termination of residents' careers – might also vary with the type of treatment approach. At the very least one might assume that defaulting rates would be greater in instrumental communities simply because the greater length of expected resident careers offers more scope for the operation of unforeseen contingencies (an unhappy love affair, committing a custodial offence, funding difficulties, and so forth) to hasten a resident's departure, but such an assumption would not be justified. Certainly some of the instrumental communities (notably the concept houses) have high defaulting rates, but most of this defaulting occurs within the first few months (see, for example, Volkman and Cressey's 1963 study of the original concept house, Synanon). However, from observations of defaulting during the fieldwork period, some of the instrumental communities in our study (Parkneuk, and the Camphill community) had relatively low proportions of defaulters and some of the reality-confronting communities (for example, Ashley) had relatively high proportions of defaulters.

We might infer that it is not an instrumental or reality-confronting approach as such that promotes high defaulting, but rather particular features of individual instrumental and reality-confronting regimes which exacerbate or protect against residents' proclivities to default; this is a topic we shall return to in our final chapter.

To summarise, assessments of residents in each individual community took different forms between the different communities, and even within the same communities the fact that assessment was a recurrent activity meant that its forms might vary considerably – for example, the co-existence of the formal clinics and the tacit agreements of co-workers at the Camphill community. The content of assessments was shaped by the content of notions of resident progress held in the different communities. Some broad similarities could be seen in the content of notions of resident progress found in communities that held similar approaches to therapeutic work. At a minimum level, all reality-confronting communities would see progress in the assimilation of residents into the culture of the community and in residents' increasing reflectivity on previously taken-for-granted patterns of behaviour, whilst all instrumental communities would judge progress by improvements in task performance.

However, we have shown that our distinction between different approaches to therapeutic work only distinguishes broad inter-community differences in assessments of residents. This is partly due to the cross-cutting influence of a further factor, namely, the differential relative strength of an orientation towards rehabilitation held across different communities. Communities with a strong orientation towards rehabilitation operated with marks of resident progress in rehabilitation following on from, and in addition to, marks of progress in treatment. The only communities with a strong rehabilitative bent which did not operate with such additional benchmarks were Beeches and the concept house – at Beeches the presence of a resident status-hierarchy was thought to move the resident automatically towards rehabilitation as the resident received promotion in the hierarchy.

A further complication was the intermediate position of the concept house. As we saw in the previous chapter, the concept house used reality-confronting techniques within an instrumental approach to therapy. Accordingly, it was no surprise to find that the concept house used both instrumental and reality-confronting techniques of resident assessment.

Finally, we saw that the particular marks of resident progress associated with each of our two treatment approaches could possibly serve to shape broad inter-community differences in patterns of resident careers, although again the picture was complicated by the cross-cutting effect of inter-community differences in orientation to rehabilitation. Yet we noted, in respect of variations in defaulting rates, that a satisfactory explanation for such variations could not be found at the broad level of instrumental versus reality-confronting differences. Rather it seems that such an explanation might be found in particular features of individual instrumental and reality-confronting regimes which served to protect against high defaulting rates. This is a subject to which we will return in the concluding chapter, where we will draw attention to particular aspects of individual community practice which, from a comparative perspective, seemed to confer special benefits in the regimes in which they were applied.

In this chapter we have concentrated upon the different ways in which different communities conceptualise resident progress. In the following chapter, by contrast, we shall concentrate upon variations in the audience for redefinitional work across our community and the residents' strategies for resisting redefinitional work.

Chapter 5
Audience and resident resistance

Introduction

We have shown that the distinction made in Chapter 3 between reality-confronting and instrumental approaches to therapy remained relevant in Chapter 4: conceptualisations of resident progress showed broad differences between communities according to whether a community pursued an instrumental or a reality-confronting approach. The same distinction in approach to therapy is relevant to our topic in this chapter, that of the audience for redefinitional work. We shall show that the typical audience for redefinitional work in instrumental communities is composed of staff, while the typical audience for redefinitional work in reality-confronting communities is composed of residents. By focusing on variations in the audience for redefinitional work we aim to draw attention to a fundamental distinction in the social organisation of therapy in therapeutic communities.

So far in our analysis we have considered the events and activities in therapeutic communities from what is arguably a staff perspective. To view everyday community events in accordance with their bearing on therapeutic work is to view those events in relation to the *staff* project. Certainly residents assist in that staff project (and indeed their assistance is indispensable) and many residents come to endorse the staff project and adopt it for their own. But prior to that endorsement, and recurrently throughout many resident careers, residents have their own projects, their own immediate and long-term aims and objectives. In the latter part of this chapter we try to correct our previous overly consensual picture of therapeutic community practice by describing the contest – the techniques of power and resistance – between staff and residents in therapeutic communities.

Audience

An audience can be defined as the hearer(s) of an utterance and can be singular or plural. Where the audience is plural not all of those who are hearers are necessarily also being addressed: some are merely copresent whilst another is the 'addressee' or 'target'. Sociolinguistics normally treats as a straightforward matter the determination of addressee within an audience – the addressee is seen to be the person being spoken to. However, ethnographic studies of speech have revealed that the selection by the speaker of the addressee is often covert, and that within the audience the position of addressee may be ambiguous and flexibly extensible. A notable example of such studies is Fisher's (1976) work on Barbadian 'dropped remarks', where a speaker uses a sham addressee in order indirectly to insult the copresent or overhearing real addressee. For example:

> A woman chose to wear an overly bright shade of lipstick to a party. She overheard a woman say, 'Oh, I thought your mouth was burst', to a man whose lips were perfectly in order. (Fisher, 1976, p. 231).

Reality-confronting communities present a further and contrasting example of audience ambiguity. Those residents in the audience who are apparently merely copresent with the addressee are expected to examine their situation to see whether there are similarities with that of the addressee. Thus the target for therapeutic talk is flexibly extensible within the audience beyond the ostensible addressee to others of those copresent. This requirement for residents to examine their situation for similarities with that of the addressee ('sharing') has been sensitively analysed by Wootton (1977). The importance for community practice of the extensibility of the target to others in the audience can be gleaned from the fact no group therapy, only one-to-one psychotherapy, would be possible if there were no perceived overlap between different residents' problems.

The extent of this fluidity of target within a therapeutic community audience can be gauged by the list below of different targets for staff and resident redefinitional work. The list is not meant to be exhaustive, merely to encompass the main differences found:

	Speaker	Primary target	Secondary target	Copresent
1	staff	resident	none	residents and staff
2	staff	resident	residents	residents and staff
3	staff	staff	residents	residents and staff
4	staff	resident	none	none
5	staff	staff	none	none
6	resident	resident	none	none
7	resident	resident	residents	residents
8	resident	resident	staff	residents and staff
9	resident	resident	residents	residents and staff

In some of these cases (notably 3 and 8) the primary target is often a 'sham' target, as with Fisher's dropped remarks. For example, a day hospital staff member cut in on another staff member's account in the community group of his troubles with his girlfriend to ask 'Why don't you take the hint to shut up?', an indirect criticism of the residents present for their failure to 'share' with the staff member.

We shall now examine the way in which the target varies and shifts between different communities, beginning with a comparison of Faswells and Camphill, and using differences between communities in aspects of the audience for redefinitional work to demonstrate associated differences in the social organisation of therapy.

Faswells

Within Faswells a good deal of emphasis was directed at providing residents with redefinitions of their activities, and shifts of addressee within an audience were a common occurrence:

> The large group. The resident chairperson asks one of the residents (Susan) why she missed the morning meeting. At first Susan refuses to answer and then, staring blankly at the floor, begins to sob. The other residents sit in silence.

SUSAN: There's no point, it's up to you anyway, it's always up to you. (Silence)

CAROLE (resident): Can't you say what is bothering you?

SUSAN: I've talked about it in my small group. To go over it again would be a waste of time. (Silence apart from Susan's sniffles)

GRAHAME (resident): Even though you might feel it would be a waste of time, can't you say how you feel? Talking about my problems helped me though at the time I didn't think it would. Just getting other people's views helped. (Silence)

MARION (staff nurse): There seems to be a lot of anger in the room today – can't we face what Susan is telling us?

GARY (resident): Yeah, what about all those effing people this morning going on about the silences in the afternoon meeting? Why don't they say something?

Gradually, the other residents join in expressing their concern and care for Susan, sharing their experiences and gently encouraging her to speak about what is upsetting her. Though she is still upset at the end of the meeting she comments that 'I've been helped by the concern you have all shown me.' The meeting is closed and I sense a feeling of achievement amongst the nurses and the residents. This has been a good meeting.

On this occasion the initial addressee for redefinitional work is Susan (with the nurse and the other residents encouraging her to say what is bothering her), the role of addressee then shifts to the resident group as a whole with the nurse's comment about there seeming to be a lot of anger in the room today, and then finally shifts back to Susan with her conclusion that she has indeed been helped by the concern the group has shown her.

Residents at Faswells were not expected to sit in the groups and await their 'turn'; they were not expected to be passively copresent while another was addressed. Instead, they were expected to monitor discussions where others were the ostensible target and inspect their own circumstances for parallels with the topic under discussion. Residents were expected, of their own volition, to view themselves as potential secondary targets for redefinitions.

To contribute to the discussions, citing parallels with one's own experiences, was known as 'sharing'. Sharing contributions were seen as performing a host of potentially therapeutic tasks: moving the discussion on from an exclusive focus on a single resident, offering 'proven' remedies for the addressee's problems, disproving the uniqueness of the addressee's difficulties, providing occasions for the description of one's feelings, and so on. So strong was the expectation that residents should make sharing contributions that the absence of any such contributions from residents could be treated rhetorically by staff as a message in itself: 'Can't we face what Susan is telling us?', 'Why don't you take the hint to shut up?' Such staff redefinitions of silences served as exhortations to residents to share, to see themselves as secondary or additional addressees in the discussion.

In addition to staff and residents providing, and in turn being provided with, redefinitions of each other's activities, a good deal of importance was attached to staff feeding back to residents an assessment of the residents' work in the groups. In the period immediately following some of the large groups, for example, staff would retire to the staff room to compose a written report that would be read out aloud to residents at the next meeting. On occasion the addressee for these accounts would be an individual resident, with the other residents being merely copresent. On other occasions the resident group as a whole would be the addressee for staff redefinitional accounts. We provide below two illustrative examples of this contrast:

> Difficult to accept and easy to forget that in reality as opposed to fantasy the responsibility for devising the community's rules belongs to everybody – residents no less than staff. Likewise, the community's pains such as those caused by having to discharge Mike (resident) are shared by everybody. It was an omission that this was not shared by a formal vote instead of silent agreement.
>
> We feel that Lesley's immediate task is to establish an independent relationship to Faswells. We draw her attention to the potentiality of her new post as chairperson. She may be able to use this role as an opportunity to develop a two-way relationship with the community. Without undermining the stability and importance of Lesley's home environment we would like to emphasise that when she experiences distress in Faswells she uses the time to work on it here rather than going home and avoiding the growth opportunity.

Although the contrast here is between those accounts which were directed at individual residents and those directed at the resident group as a whole, in fact the distinction is more apparent than real since, in reading these reports out loud to the meeting at large, even those reports targeted at individual residents would take on something of a collective significance. Indeed such reports often stood as one way in which staff sought to structure fellow residents' 'seeing' in relation to individual residents. So, for example, the advice given to Lesley that she use the meetings to work out her anxieties, rather than returning home when she was upset, was meant for her *and* the group, since it stood as one way of advising the group that they pay particular attention to this aspect of Lesley's behaviour and confront her when it was clear to them that she was indeed returning home in preference to using the meetings.

Although within the group meetings, residents were expected to see themselves as the target for each other's disclosures, to listen to what other residents were saying, examine their own situation in the light of these comments, and respond in kind, there were occasions when, for one reason or another, residents refused or were unable to comply with this expectation. At such times staff would often explicitly select from the range of copresent residents an individual who they thought ought to have been able to respond to another resident's comments and directly invite a comment. In this way staff could be seen making explicit use of the extensibility of the target within an audience to develop and broaden the therapeutic discussion of residents' activities. This is apparent in the example below:

> Large group. Eileen (resident) comments that she saw Ivor (resident) going off on his own obviously pretty angry. Arthur (resident) asks Ivor if he was angry about the custard (apparently the previous evening residents on the cooking rota had failed to collect the custard from the kitchens). Ivor remains sitting in silence and Clare (resident) comments that she, like Ivor, feels as if people are no longer caring much about each other. The meeting lapses into silence until Sally (nurse) turns to Richard (resident) and comments 'You, Richard, felt something similar last week, didn't you?' At first Richard merely shrugs his shoulders in a 'couldn't care less' manner. Philip (resident) then accuses Richard of being one of the most uncaring members on the ward and instances how at dinner this afternoon he finished off the remaining sausages before other residents had collected their first helping.

Here, although the discussion starts with Ivor as the target, his failure to respond is repaired by Clare who comments that she too feels the community is becoming more uncaring. The meeting at this point lapses into silence and it appears that none of the other residents is prepared to enter into the discussion; it is perhaps as much for this reason as any other that Sally, the nurse, actually invites a response from one of the other residents whom she knows to be of a similar opinion to both Ivor and Clare. By changing the addressee in this way Sally is able to continue a discussion which at one point looked as if it was going to come to a premature close as a result of residents' unwillingness to examine their own situation for parallels with that of Ivor.

Despite the fact that residents were the typical addressee or target for staff discussions of their activities, there were occasions when this was not the case and where staff would exchange redefinitional accounts only amongst themselves. One situation in which this would occur was where staff were attempting to produce a consensual case picture of individual residents:

> Staff meeting. Michael (consultant) raises the matter of Alan (resident) who he says is being increasingly disruptive in meetings. Karen (psychiatrist) comments that staff are scapegoating Alan (a member of her small group) by referring to him as a frightened and nasty individual. The consultant at this point responds by saying that Alan is a frightened and nasty individual and that staff should be careful not to allow him to sabotage the structure of the community by, for example, turning up late for meetings, messing around in meetings, and attempting to prolong the meetings beyond the agreed closing time.

Another situation in which Faswells staff would exchange such accounts only amongst themselves was where the individual residents concerned were seen to have reached a saturation point where further confrontational work was held to be of little or no benefit. As one of the Faswells nurses put it 'the time for talking is long gone, now there's only one thing left – action – and that, for most of them, is moving out.' Although certain of the Faswells staff held this to be the case for some residents, it was noticeable that they would often continue to redefine those residents' activities in their own meetings though without providing the residents concerned with a similar redefinition.

Relatedly, there was also a certain wariness on the part of some of the Faswells nurses about interpreting residents' activities in the absence of the psychiatrists. At such times nurses would exchange comments about residents in their own meetings, in preference to making the residents themselves the audience for their redefinitions. McKeganey recorded the following conversation, for example, in the staff room immediately following one of the large group meetings organised by the nurses:

STAFF NURSE: Did you see anything about Rebecca in the meeting?
NM: She was nervous, fiddling, that's all.
STAFF NURSE: With the towel.
NM: What do you mean?
STAFF NURSE: Did you not see the way she was holding the towel, rocking it close to her chest, as if it were a child? . . . I nodded to you for confirmation.
NM: Why didn't you mention it at the meeting?
STAFF NURSE: I didn't know how she might react and anyway she may have gone over it in her small group. Maybe I was wrong about that. That's why I looked at you and to you, Mike (charge nurse). If you had confirmed it I would have said something.

To summarise, within Faswells staff adopted a reality-confronting approach to therapy in which particular importance was attached to making residents the audience for redefinitional accounts of their activities. Although residents certainly were the typical audience for these accounts, there were situations where staff judged it more appropriate to exchange these accounts only amongst themselves. The situation at Camphill as regards the typical audience for redefinitional work was, as we shall see, the opposite of that in Faswells.

Camphill

Within Camphill the audience for redefinitional work was determined by a backstage/frontstage division wherein explicit reference to therapeutic matters in the company of the children was generally eschewed (McKeganey, 1983). This was very evident to McKeganey early on in his fieldwork when, in the company of a group of children, he innocently enquired about a forthcoming 'college meeting' to discuss the problems of one particular child. The co-worker on this occasion ushered him into one of the side-rooms and commented: 'The first thing is: never mention the child's name when other children are around. You never know who is listening and they have ears everywhere.'

Perhaps the clearest example of this backstage restriction of therapeutic discussion of the children's activities occurred in relation to the formal clinics, where, although the children would be present for a part of the time (the physical examination), they would always be shown out of the room before the adults had begun to discuss their situation in detail:

> During the clinic today one of the children showed a marked reluctance to enter the room, only doing so after much coaxing and cajoling from the dormitory parent and even then maintaining an odd catatonic-like posture throughout the examination. After a few moments the doctor concluded his examination and commented, 'A real first class performance ... very nice ... good ... you can go and get dressed now, put on your shoes ... it was nice seeing you. I do think you are really getting much better ... good, that's it ... fine, off you go. (Child exits.) That of course is really pure hysteria.'
> HOUSEMOTHER: Now?
> DOCTOR: Yes.

It was not, however, simply material bearing on the formal clinics and college meetings that would be restricted to the backstage. In an earlier chapter we commented on the way in which Camphill staff held it to be very important to combine a range of different handicaps in each house so as to make use of the help differently handicapped children could offer each other. Staff did not, however, leave to chance the possibility of such relationships of mutual help developing between the children but adopted a kind of benevolent social engineering approach in which they consciously sought to bring about dormitory partnerships or dinner table partnerships with this end in mind:

> Coffee room discussion amongst the co-workers who, apart from planning various activities, are considering the relationships between the children.

ELLEN (co-worker): I think it's a good idea for Mary to sit on Karen's table. She was very helpful with Steven (child) this afternoon, very knowledgeable, talking about what Susan (previous dormitory parent) used to do.

PETRA (houseparent): Susan used to say though that Mary was a bit overbearing.

ELLEN: Yes, she really wants to pull him right away and spoon-feed him. Still, at the moment she can be quite a help.

This social engineering work was also restricted to the backstage, exchanged only amongst the adult co-workers, thereby leaving the children largely unaware of the way in which their relationships with one another were the subject of detailed staff planning and monitoring.

Despite the fact that staff operated a strict backstage/frontstage division in the therapeutic discussions of childrens' activities, it was not the case that co-workers coming fresh to the house were immediately provided with large areas of backstage knowledge about the children. Rather, it was left largely up to the individual co-workers themselves to work out their own relationships with the children. One of the Camphill houseparents commented:

> The most important influence on the new co-workers is their meeting with the child, and developing a sense of knowing when the child is doing something because she is misbehaving and when she is doing something because this is her illness.

Although senior staff would, occasionally, provide junior co-workers with backstage advice as to how certain children ought to be related to, that advice would tend to be in the typically abbreviated form of suggestions as to what would be 'good' for specific children. Whilst the staff group as a whole would have access to the formal information held on the children, contained, for example, in the house notes, in fact there was relatively little emphasis placed on staff pooling their knowledge about the children within the staff group as a whole.

While the audience and target for redefinitional work at Camphill tended to be staff, there were occasions, as there were at Faswells, where the opposite would occur and where the children would be made aware of the therapeutic purpose behind a staff member's intervention. At such times the children themselves would be cast in the audience, or target, role:

> This evening I sat in as Karla (dormitory parent) settled her dormitory. As a final thing she held hands with each child individually and ran through one of the anthroposophical prayers. I was intrigued as to what she would do with Diane – an elective mute. In fact what happened was that Karla said all the words and Diane made a kind of singing noise in time with Karla's recitation. I noticed that each of the other children watched intently throughout all this and when Karla moved to the next child one of the other girls piped up, 'She's getting better at it, Karla! When subsequently I told Karla how impressed I had been by the whole thing she commented that it was good for the other girls to see how hard Diane would try to say the prayer.

It is important to stress that the other children here were not simply copresent at the Karla/Diane interaction, but rather the interaction was at least in part staged for their benefit. That the dormitory parent on this occasion made quite a thing of running through the prayer with Diane was not simply because this was held to be beneficial for Diane, but also because it was held to be beneficial for the other children to see how hard Diane tried to say the prayer despite her handicap. Both Diane and the other children, then, were the target for the dormitory parent's intervention.

Similarly, there were occasions when, with certain children, at certain times, staff judged it appropriate to relax the backstage/frontstage division and openly provide the children with the sorts of accounts of their activities that would be more commonly heard within those communities adopting a reality-confronting approach to therapy:

> This evening Stephanie (dormitory parent) explained to me how she felt it was very important to spend some time each evening with Pauline (child) discussing the various things that had happened during the day and her reactions to them. Stephanie explained that part of Pauline's difficulties was in understanding where she stood in relation to things that happened around her and that this was one way in which she could develop such an understanding.

Despite the overall emphasis at Camphill on restricting the therapeutic discussion of the children's activities to the backstage, there were occasions when individual children themselves would be the target for these accounts.

So far in this chapter we have used the contrasting examples of Faswells and Camphill to show how the typical audience for redefinitional work varied according to whether the approach to therapy adopted was of the reality-confronting or instrumental kind. Once again, however, we are dealing with a difference in emphasis rather than an absolute difference in kind, since there were occasions at Faswells when staff alone were the audience for redefinitional work and there were occasions at Camphill when the audience was comprised of children. In the remainder of this part of the chapter we shall concentrate on the question of audience in relation to our other communities, starting first with those adopting a reality-confronting approach to therapy.

The other communities

Despite the fact that it was residents who were the typical audience for redefinitional accounts at Ravenscroft, there were occasions when staff operated a similar backstage/frontstage division to that found at Camphill, and certain topics were discussed only amongst themselves. One of these had to do with clinical discussions of residents' diagnoses. During the fieldwork at Ravenscroft, for example, staff frequently discussed the case of one resident (Gary) in their closed meetings. Apparently Gary had given staff cause for concern after having explained his reluctance to speak in the formal groups by noting to one of the nurses that he often knew in advance what people were going to say, and that anyway he felt very uncomfortable knowing that people were discussing him. When this conversation was recounted in the staff meeting there was general concern as to whether Gary might be suffering from some kind of psychotic illness that could be exacerbated by the techniques of group therapy. As a result of this speculation staff were enjoined to 'keep an eye on Gary' and to note any other significant signs of a psychotic condition. No mention was made of confronting Gary about this aspect of his behaviour, rather it was seen as something which staff ought to decide for themselves without bringing it to either Gary's or the group's attention.

The tendency to restrict explicit discussion of clinical matters to the backstage was also evident at the day hospital. Bloor recorded the following fieldnote, which reports on a similar situation to that at Ravenscroft:

> In the staff group Dave (nurse) deferred to the clinical staff on a matter of psychiatry. I've heard nursing staff deferring to the clinical staff on such matters as medication and physical illness but this was the first time I'd heard the nurses defer on such a matter. He asked Alan and Simon (psychiatrists) whether from their experience they'd say to confront Wanda might push her into a psychosis. Alan agreed that it was a risk but thought the chance had to be taken.

Despite the fact that on this occasion staff did indeed decide to confront Wanda, it is perhaps significant that they opted to raise the clinical pros and cons of such a move in their own meeting away from the patients.

In addition to restricting the discussion of more overtly clinical matters to the backstage, there was a further parallel between the day hospital, Faswells and Ravenscroft in that staff also restricted to the backstage their attempts at generating a consensual case picture about individual residents' difficulties.

Staff in the day hospital also recognised occasions when it would be counter-therapeutic for them to work through their feelings in the patient groups. At such times staff were encouraged to hold back from speaking in the patient groups, and to work through their feelings of anger or frustration, for example, in their own closed meetings:

> In the review group Clive (consultant) returned again to the theme of the informal patient culture. I recapitulated my remarks on the visit-to-Maggie affair. Clive remarked that I was probably resenting the remarks made about patients in the review group. (True – I'd said so to other staff in his absence that I had found it difficult listening to the cutting remarks on Steve's (patient) decision to get a job as a barman). Clive pointed out, however, that the staff group was also a therapeutic group and that there were times when it was inappropriate for staff to express their feelings in the large group – they had to be suppressed and then let out in the staff group.

That staff in the day hospital were restricting quite a few of their accounts of residents' activities to the backstage was made apparent to Bloor when he switched from spending most of his time with patients to spending more time with staff. As a result of this switch Bloor suddenly became aware of how discrepant his view of certain patients was from that held by staff in their own closed meetings:

> I was forcefully struck in the staff group by the discrepancy in the staff's view of Martin (patient) and my own. His every action seemed to be reinterpreted in an unfavourable light: he had left the day hospital at the weekend to stay with friends prior to moving into a bed-and-breakfast until he could get into a flat with an ex-patient. He was seen on the steps of the day hospital at shortly after 9 (though the group doesn't start until 10.15) conversing with some of the in-patients. Earlier he had been prowling about the wards looking for a razor. All this was seen as evidence of his dependence on the day hospital. (Why couldn't he shave at his friends', for Chrissake? Don't they have electricity?) Innocuous explanations were not considered ... Later in the day I tried to give Martin credit for the work he did with other patients ... but John (staff) got rather angry and called him a 'salesman', asked what had happened to his anger, and called him irresponsible ... It's possible of course that Martin has conned me but the strength of feeling about him seemed a little disproportionate. I was reminded of another patient who staff seemed to scapegoat in their groups while I was doing pilot work.

The extent of this discrepancy between Bloor's impression of certain patients and that held by staff in their own closed meetings is particularly interesting since it gives some indication of the degree to which, even within a situation in which a good deal of importance is attached to making residents the audience for redefinitions of their activities, there will still be many occasions when these redefinitions are exchanged only amongst staff.

Within Ashley, the extent to which residents were to be the audience for staff redefinitions of their activities was very much a topical concern during the fieldwork, in keeping with each of the reality-confronting communities included in our study. Although Ashley residents were the typical audience for redefinitional accounts of their activities, there were certain areas of the Ashley programme to which residents did not have access and where the audience for staff accounts were staff themselves. During the fieldwork, for example, there were discussions about allowing residents access to staff meetings and resident files. Although the house warden was not averse to 'democratising' the Ashley programme in this way there was a feeling amongst some other staff that both of these moves could present problems:

> Staff meeting: some discussion of a previous suggestion to open up part of the staff meeting to the rest of the community. Dave explained that this had arisen partly because of resident resentment/interest in the meeting (what do you talk about in there?) and partly through a staff feeling that they should be more open.... It was suggested that the finance/residents' fees part of the meeting should be open but that referrals and resident review should remain closed. Frank said that the resident review *could* be open but it would probably, for the residents, only mean them going over ground they had already covered in counselling sessions. Later he repeated that the resident reviews could be open but it would need a lot of staff courage. I took him to mean that staff would find it difficult to be as open and honest about their feelings concerning residents in an open meeting as they are in the present closed staff meeting. The matter is to be given further thought.

When this matter was subsequently raised it was decided that although individual residents *could* have access to the staff reviews, they ought only to have access to those parts of the review which referred directly to them. In practice this would have involved such a constant ferrying of residents into and out of the room that staff judged it to be impracticable. As far as residents' access to files was concerned, again there was a feeling that access should only be granted for the resident to see his or her own file and this should only cover items which staff had written during the resident's stay in the house. Ashley staff maintained that it woulds be unethical to allow residents access to, for example, referral letters that had originally been written in the belief that their contents would not be revealed to residents. It was judged to be inappropriate to provide the resident group as a whole with the sort of information which was currently shared by the staff group as a whole. In relation to these two areas of extended access, audience was seen in individual rather than group terms.

Having reviewed the situation of audience in relation to our remaining reality-confronting communities we turn now to those where the approach was more instrumental: Beeches, Parkneuk, and the concept house.

Although, like Camphill, Beeches also adopted an instrumental approach to therapy, there were striking differences between the two communities in the audience for redefinitional work – particularly in relation to the pooling of information amongst the staff group. At Camphill, for example, relatively little emphasis was placed on staff sharing interpretive accounts of the children's activities; rather, individual staff were encouraged to work out their own relationship with individual children in order to create a situation where different staff had a different relationship with the same child. At Beeches, by contrast, a great deal of importance was attached to staff having the same view and acting in a like manner to each resident. These backstage efforts at developing a consensual staff case picture, and a consistent staff approach, were exemplified by the staff 'Intervention Book', which would list separately for each resident the approved form of staff intervention:

> Staff meeting. Lengthy discussion of Tina and her reversion to uncooperative behaviour in the programme. Lisa said that she still seemed attracted to the idea of a passive, institutionalised life: unlike many of the other residents, she had no enthusiasm for the idea of eventually getting a flat of her own. I said I was unhappy that by her non-cooperation she was forcing the staff into taking all the decisions for her ... Jean suggested that in such situations we present her non-cooperation as a decision in itself, one option among others, and one which would have consequences (preferably short-term) for her. Lisa said that would be an 'informative' intervention; Kim duly entered it in the Intervention Book.

The instrumental approach to therapy, the programming of residents' activities, was facilitated by making the staff group as a whole the primary target for redefinitional work.

While it was generally the case that staff were the typical audience within instrumental communities for redefinitions, the situation at Parkneuk was rather different. Redefinitional work at Parkneuk involving staff or residents occurred only infrequently. In fact, the situation in this respect was somewhat similar to that at Camphill, since in both communities staff aimed to create a foster family-like environment around the residents in which it would have been seen as wholly inappropriate and very disruptive to continually provide them with redefinitions of their situation. At Camphill, however, formal assessments of the children were made even if these were regarded as items of backstage knowledge. At Parkneuk, by contrast, the backstage/frontstage division was much less clearly expressed because of the rarity of even these formal assessments. As we have already seen, therapeutically oriented discussions of resident's activities at Parkneuk tended to be highly abbreviated – often assuming a form such as 'It would be really good to take Victor (withdrawn schizophrenic) camping.' It was only on very rare occasions that Parkneuk staff would provide the residents with redefinitions of their behaviour. Even amongst themselves, staff showed a reluctance to interpret residents' activities. Parkneuk staff, then, were in no way concerned to act with anything like the one voice of the Beeches staff, but rather maintained the importance of different adults having different relationships with the same child:

> Megan (staff) points out that different staff can behave differently to the same resident ... I realise that this is indeed the Parkneuk method: all staff interact with all residents, although each resident probably has one staff member who is especially close to them, and different staff do play different roles with the same resident. This is not a uniform pattern since some staff play more than one role with the same resident and the partial closure surrounding therapeutic contexts (the house, the field) means that staff members must occasionally switch roles because the appropriate staff actor is missing.

The audience at Parkneuk was an individual (singular) one, a matter of individual relationships between staff and residents, even if within those relationships there was very little explicit discussion of therapy as a topical concern in itself.

Lastly in this section we have the concept house. To talk of a staff-resident split in the audience for redefinitional work in the concept house is itself something of an oversimplification since staff appointed senior residents to supervisory positions in the house 'structure', and since many of the staff were themselves ex-addicts. Nevertheless, Fonkert was aware of a similar backstage/frontstage division to that which was evident in a number of our other communities. Junior residents were excluded from staff meetings, for example, but some of the senior residents were sometimes required to attend. Fonkert noticed, however, that on those occasions when senior residents attended the staff groups there was a noticeable shift in the tenor of the discussions. When he asked senior staff members about this it was pointed out that with the attendance of residents the staff meetings would take on a more therapeutic orientation, and attention would be directed to whether the senior residents could keep the confidences to which they had been given access as a result of their attendance at the staff meeting. Staff would retain a separate agenda, even on those occasions when they opened their meetings up to senior residents.

We noted in Chapter 4 the importance which concept house staff attached to behavioural conformity, and the assiduity with which they looked for signs of that conformity. Although Fonkert was not ideally placed to identify specific instances of residents 'conning' staff, he was aware of residents, on occasion, making remarks to each other that were principally intended to signal such a conformity to staff, whilst the residents concerned privately maintained their own discrepant or agnostic viewpoints (see also the silent scepticism that accompanied Tony Morrelli's conformity at the Zeta concept house, described in Gould et al., 1974).

Finally, staff in the concept house had devised a mechanism for communicating aspects of the residents' activities to the community as a whole that was somewhat analogous to the staff 'report back' employed at Faswells. Concept house residents were sometimes required to wear a signboard signalling to the community as a whole their transgressions of house rules ('I have brought the values of the street into the house'). Whilst it may be thought that the wearing of these signboards had a punitive function, in fact they were seen by staff as providing an opportunity for further redefinitional work since individuals would be expected to explain their boards in the formal groups.

Recapitulation

We have sought to show here the way in which the typical audience or target for redefinitional work varied across our communities, depending upon whether the approach to therapy that was adopted was of the reality-confronting or instrumental kind. Within our reality-confronting communities – Faswells, Ravenscroft, the day hospital, and Ashley – the typical audience for redefinitional work was the residents. In each of these communities, however, 'audience' was a flexibly extensible concept, and shifts within audience between those who were the target and those who were merely copresent were very evident. Similarly, despite the fact that residents were the typical audience for redefinitions, there were occasions in each of these communities when such accounts were exchanged only amongst the staff.

Within those communities adopting an instrumental approach to therapy – Camphill, Beeches, Parkneuk and the concept house – it was staff who were the typical audience for redefinitions. Once again, however, there were occasions within each of these communities when the residents themselves would be the audience for these accounts.

In communities of both broad types, however, one could find evidence of a backstage/frontstage division in the discussion of certain material that was held to be very important in the social organisation of therapy.

So far in this study we have considered the therapeutic process within our communities from what is arguably a staff perspective and have largely glossed over the extent to which residents were able to challenge staff accounts of their activities. Since we would not wish to be charged with presenting an overly consensual picture of life within a therapeutic community we shall now concentrate on the related topics of power, surveillance, and resident resistance.

Power, surveillance and resident resistance

The conceptual approach to power that we shall follow here is that associated with the work of Michel Foucault (see especially Foucault, 1980). According to Foucault, power is not a property, or an attribute of a given social status, but a strategic relationship; power exists in its exercise. The exemplar for such an approach is Foucault's study of the philosopher Jeremy Bentham's design for a model prison, the Panopticon (Foucault, 1977; Foucault, 1980). According to Bentham, the best way to control and reform a prison population with a minimum of warders was to create a situation in which the prisoners felt themselves to be under constant surveillance, thus the Panopticon involved an arrangement of cells centrifugally placed around a central observatory. The prisoner's openness to surveillance was thought to lead to dissuasion and ultimately reform: 'it is necessary for the inmate to be ceaselessly under the eyes of an inspector; this is to lose the power and even almost the idea of wrong-doing.' (Bentham quoted in Foucault, 1980, p. 154).

Foucault linked the exemplary Panopticon with his earlier analysis of the new language of seeing that, he maintained, had its birth in the Paris clinics of the late eighteenth century. This new language of seeing constructed the body as an invariate biological reality and laid the foundations for modern medical knowledge (Armstrong, 1983). In these pioneer clinics a new strategic relationship was evident between an individualised body and a disembodied gaze – the clinical gaze. The exercise of surveillance in the clinical gaze constituted a power relationship within the therapeutic encounter.

Although in his later work Foucault de-emphasised the modern importance of surveillance as a technique of power, there are good grounds for supposing that within therapeutic communities, at least, surveillance remains as salient as ever. At the outset of this book we defined the therapeutic community approach in terms of the redefinition of activities in the light of a therapeutic paradigm, with the nature of that paradigm shifting from one community to the next. Yet before an event, activity, or utterance can be redefined in this way it first has to be perceived. Surveillance, therefore, is a logical prerequisite for the kind of redefinitional work that we have suggested is the very basis of the therapeutic community approach.

It is possible to identify different techniques of surveillance associated with our two broad types of community. Within those communities adopting a reality-confronting approach to therapy, surveillance tends to be both pervasive and naturalistic – pervasive in the sense that *all* resident behaviour has to be potentially open to surveillance for confrontation to occur, and naturalistic in the sense that residents have to feel relatively uninhibited by the fact of being observed. It is for these reasons that surveillance tends to be normally subsumed under other activities – cleaning the house, washing dishes, watching television – with the associated work of confrontation often being postponed to one of the formal group meetings. In Ashley one of the staff members brought his dirty washing with him when he was on night duty in order to have a plausible reason for repeatedly going back and forth through the community's public rooms, supposedly checking on the progress of his washing, but in reality monitoring residents' activities. In concealing from residents the real reason for his actions the staff member was able to employ a disembodied gaze – disembodied in the sense that his monitoring of residents was carried out surreptitiously and was more penetrative for that reason. Had residents been alerted to this strategy they would, of course, have been able to take some kind of remedial action.

Behaviour that was judged to be significant, in signalling either residents' difficulties or their progress, would be communicated to other staff in Ashley by being recorded in the log-book or by being discussed at the next meeting. In this way the staff gaze was further disembodied since it became a collective gaze, unattributable to any single individual. Knowledge about individual residents would cease to be a matter of what any one staff member knew about that person and would become instead part of the common stock of knowledge held collectively amongst staff.

Non-residential communities like the day hospital, or those that were only partially residential, like Ravenscroft, clearly face difficulties in maintaining the desired level of surveillance. Staff in both of these communities could often be heard exhorting residents to bring back to the groups material on events that occurred outside the formal programme and could be seen thereby to be artificially extending the surveillance of residents' activities beyond the boundaries of the institution.

Surveillance within instrumental communities tended to be more a matter of formal supervision. Residents' activities were often tightly controlled in time and space, with restrictions being placed in the concept house, for example, on new residents contacting any individuals outside the community. Surveillance in some of these communities was further facilitated by incorporating residents into a formal hierarchy with associated rights and privileges and charging them with the responsibility of monitoring each other's activities.

The importance of surveillance in relations of power in both types of communities was apparent in the fact that, although techniques of resident resistance took many forms in each of the communities studied here, the most frequently observed forms of resistance were directed against surveillance. However, before focusing upon the residents' techniques for limiting the surveillance of their activities, we shall look first at certain other, less widespread, forms of resistance, namely collective ideological dissent, contested redefinitions, non-cooperation, and escape. In a final section we shall examine some of the staff strategies for countering these techniques of resident resistance.

Collective ideological dissent

By collective ideological dissent we mean an articulated counter-culture opposed in principle and in practice to the staff project and aimed at capturing the community as a locale for its own project. By definition, such ideological dissent is very visible, but apart from one possible instance no such resistance was observed in any of our communities. The one possible exception occurred during Bloor's pilot study at the day hospital and had to do with the weekly evening social club set up by an attached social worker. Some of the patients expressed the view that care was more readily available in the socials than in the formal groups and some staff complained that the effectiveness of the groups was being diminished by some patients' preference for speaking in the socials. However, by the time Bloor began his main period of fieldwork new patients had ceased to attend the socials.

A more certain example of ideological dissent is provided by Sharp in his study of a halfway house community (Sharp, 1975). Sharp noted the presence of a dissident clique of residents within the house who would persistently attempt to turn the group discussions into attacks on staff, the rules, 'the system', and who wished to turn the house away from its rehabilitative role and convert the community into an intentional commune which would allow more self-actualisation for residents than outside society would permit.

Contested redefinitions

A much more commonly heard technique of resident resistance had to do with specific and individual complaints. Within those communities adopting a reality-confronting approach to therapy staff redefinitions were a common locus for this kind of dissent. McKeganey recorded the following exchange in one of the Faswells large groups:

DR GRAHAM: There seem to be a lot of members absent from this meeting.

PAULA (resident): Michael has a job interview. Steven is working, I don't know about Rachel.

DR GRAHAM: Is there in these absences, which have been happening for some time now, a sense of things being unbearable, a feeling of needing to be away from these meetings?

PAULA: I don't think so, it's unavoidable if people are going to be involved in working and leaving that some of the meetings are going to have a poor attendance.

Non-cooperation

As a form of resistance non-cooperation needs little comment. It was commonly found within both types of community, though it would take different forms in each: silence in the groups, or absence from them, in the reality-confronting communities; non-participation in some of the activities in the instrumental communities. McKeganey recorded the following example of resident non-cooperation in one of the Faswells large groups:

Sharon (chairperson) opens the meeting noting that the only item on the agenda is a discussion of the rules for day membership. Before this topic can be introduced, however, one of the psychiatrists intervenes suggesting that the community should discuss the 'incident' that occurred last night. The meeting lapses into silence until another psychiatrist intervenes.

PSYCHIATRIST: We can't just sit here in silence – Graham, you know what went on, so why don't you tell us?

GRAHAM (resident): I've talked about it in my small group ... I've got nothing to say about it ... (silence)

CLIVE (nurse): What is the big secret about all this; why is it so difficult to talk about it? Can't you see how uneasy it makes everyone feel, not talking about it?

GRAHAM: Martin (ex-member) and this guy had a fight, they'd been drinking.

PSYCHIATRIST: Why was Martin here?

GRAHAM: He came in with a message.

PSYCHIATRIST: What message?

GRAHAM: I'm not going to say.

PSYCHIATRIST: Look, if you're not going to say then we are going to have to assume, and I'd stake my life it had to do with alcohol, drugs and all the excitement that goes with that.

GRAHAM: It did not.

PSYCHIATRIST: I think we are going to have to take a serious look

> at the value of residents visiting the alcohol unit. We don't know what goes on there.

Non-cooperation was normally a matter of individual resistance. However, McKeganey recorded a number of occasions in one of the reality-confronting communities when groups of residents boycotted certain of the meetings: the afternoon large groups organised by the nurses, the weekly art therapy sessions and the music therapy sessions. Similarly, Bloor observed two instances in one of the instrumental communities when some residents boycotted the weekly community meeting, and then two days later a smaller group initially refused to take part in the morning workgroup.

Escape

None of these communities was a secure institution with physical barriers to inhibit resistance in the form of departure. Nevertheless, departure, without the aid and agreement of staff, was no easy matter. Four of the communities had resident populations of adolescents, many of whom had a long background of institutionalised dependence, and who were a long way from home with only a hazy knowledge of local geography and limited funds. Despite this, McKeganey was aware of a number of reported escapes of residents from neighbouring houses in the Camphill community and Bloor noted that successful or attempted resident escapes averaged around one a month during his fieldwork at Ashley and Beeches. Considerable ingenuity was sometimes displayed in effecting these escapes. One resident, for example, hung about outside the house to intercept the postman and obtain his social security payment before catching an inter-city bus.

Unauthorised departure from the day hospital may at first sight seem a much easier task. In fact, the reality was very different. To anticipate our argument somewhat, resistance provokes counter-action: would-be defaulting patients who stayed away from the day hospital would frequently find themselves receiving a delegation of fellow-patients, who would attempt to persuade them to return. Few defaulters were proof against such persuasion and so those who were determined to leave had either to state their intention of leaving in the formal groups or resort to subterfuge: one successful defaulter refused to answer his door and another left the country.

Concealment

We turn now to the residents' strategies for limiting the surveillance of their activities. One way in which this would be achieved was through residents straightforwardly removing themselves from the scrutiny of staff. Bloor recorded the following extract, which is illustrative of this strategy:

> I was designated the staff 'group member' today (that is, the member of staff designated to work in one of the resident workgroups). I was working with Terry and Nigel in the kitchen and craft room. The work had been going reasonably well apart from an altercation between Nigel and Nancy through the craft room window but when Terry's sidekick (Roger) showed up he sloped off. I called him back and Terry lost his temper ... He tried to argue his way out of it: he was the group-leader – he had a right to go off ... so I argued back: as group-leader he couldn't go off without telling me, his fellow worker; we should finish the kitchen before we went to help Ken ... eventually he calmed down and I carried the day.

This same fieldnote extract also illustrates a related resident strategy, that of contesting staff surveillance, albeit here within the established conventions of the community workgroup. Generally these attempts at contesting staff surveillance were carried out by individual residents, though on one occasion, in Beeches, residents collectively argued for a 'residents' private room', where staff would have to knock and request admittance – thus mirroring the procedure residents had to go through in gaining access to the staff office. Staff, however, felt that such a move smacked of exclusivity and the suggestion was turned down (see Chapter 7).

Another form of concealment involved residents affecting a superficial conformity with staff expectations while simultaneously maintaining non-conformist aspirations and gratifications. Such forms of institutionalised adaptation have of course been widely reported elsewhere, for example, in Goffman's analysis of the 'secondary adjustments' seen amongst psychiatric hospital patients (Goffman, 1968). We noted earlier in this chapter Fonkert's suspicion that at least some of the comments from residents in the concept house were of this order, that is, aimed at convincing staff of a greater degree of behavioural change than had actually occurred.

Similarly, Bloor recorded the following instance during his fieldwork at Beeches:

> I said I would work with Terry today in the workgroup (I was group member) because of the events of yesterday morning's meeting when Lisa (staff) confronted him about his poor performance working outside. I noticed that when I worked alongside him (sweeping the drive) he worked very hard but when we divided the tasks he did the bare minimum. Also the work that he did do gave the maximum cosmetic effect for the resident chairman's inspection.

Relatedly, in reality-confronting communities it is sometimes possible to hear staff describe some residents as merely going through the motions of group therapy – having a practised grasp of the conventions and the argot of group work but using this familiarity as a resource to avoid expressing their 'real' feelings and problems.

A further technique for inhibiting the penetration of the staff gaze involved residents stressing the secret character of their shared knowledge:

> Sitting at table waiting for tea to be served with five residents. One of them began to talk about some incident that had occurred the other night. She was cut short by another who said 'There's only four people sitting around this table who know about that.' Tom said, 'I didn't know anything about it.' 'No, and you're not going to either.' I was the sixth.

However, it was not the case that in maintaining this level of concealment residents were constantly having to stress the secret character of their information about each other. Rather, in their interaction with each other, residents became unwitting parties to the shared knowledge of the in-group. Much of this knowledge was tacit and taken for granted (for example, who was sexually attracted to whom) and never attained the form of an explicit statement that would carry a 'secret' tag. Confidences were sustained much more naturalistically than any reference to a 'no-grassing' convention would suggest.

Counteraction

Strategies of resident resistance were, by and large, transitory in their appearance. One reason for this was the continual resident turnover. Another reason was the operation of staff strategies for counteraction.

Some counteraction was local in the sense that the forms it took varied with the form of resident resistance and varied from community to community. Thus non-cooperation would be tolerated for a period in the permissive environment of a reality-confronting community but would find a quick response in an instrumental community. In Chapter 3 we described the use of what staff in Beeches described as the 'listen technique' for overcoming the non-cooperation of one particular resident. To write of countering resident resistance in those communities characterised by their permissive environments might, at first sight, seem rather odd. However, permissiveness is never total; it is always subject to limits and qualification (see Morrice, 1965). In reality-confronting communities counteraction is frequently not a staff but a *resident* response. Just as it was fellow residents who policed the structure of activities within the concept house, so in the day hospital it was fellow patients who visited would-be defaulting patients.

Counteraction is not, however, always successful. So, for example, at Faswells there was a lingering reluctance on the part of certain nurses to confront the behaviour of 'awkward' residents. Thus one of the Faswells staff nurses explained his reluctance to interpret residents' activities in the large group in the following way:

> I confronted Caroline once and a big argument followed. When there are just the two of you (nurses) on it's easy for them to argue back and reject what you are saying. When the consultant is there they do not do that.

Techniques of counteraction could, in fact, have the effect of strengthening resident resistance. However, to the extent that counteraction is successful in defeating resident resistance then the most effective techniques of resistance will be those aimed at concealment, since their very nature ensures that staff are unlikely to know they are occurring and are thus unable to launch a response.

While staff may be unaware of specific instances of concealment, they may be well aware of the likelihood of it developing and may adopt preventive measures to stop it occurring. In the reality-confronting communities staff may continually stress the importance of 'open communications' to the successful operation of the community and the destructive potential of secretive pair-bonds. Likewise, in some instrumental communities like the concept house, secondary adjustments might be prevented by the device of the periodic 'tight house' where privileges would be revoked, duties changed and penalties increased (see Sugarman, 1974).

Summary

This chapter has been about two things: the question of who the audience for redefinitional work in our communities is, and, the question of resident resistance. At the outset of the chapter we noted that within therapeutic communities, audience is a flexibly extensible concept. This flexibility was most apparent in those communities adopting a reality-confronting approach to therapy, in which residents were expected to see themselves as the potential target for many redefinitions ostensibly directed towards others. Whilst the audience in these communities was typically composed of residents, there were also occasions when the staff were the sole audience for redefinitional work.

The situation in those communities adopting an instrumental approach to therapy was rather different. Audience in these settings was typically composed of staff with residents only relatively rarely being seen as the target for redefinitional work. In an earlier chapter we commented on how therapeutic work within instrumental communities tended to be hidden from residents; certainly much of the staff planning of the residents' activities in these communities occurred backstage.

In the second half of this chapter we concentrated upon the various means by which various residents attempted to avoid or resist the interpretive reworking of their activities. Although there was a good deal of variation in the techniques of resident resistance across our communities, the most commonly found forms of resistance were directed towards concealment from staff surveillance. Finally, we described some of the strategies staff (and fellow residents) would employ in an attempt to counteract local techniques of resident resistance.

In the following chapter we shall consider the extent to which the environment of the therapeutic community may be seen to have an impact upon the redefinitional process.

Chapter 6

The impact of the external environment

Introduction

In each of the previous chapters we have concentrated upon aspects of the therapeutic process *within* communities and have largely glossed over the extent to which these processes may be influenced by factors *outside* the community. Nevertheless, it is self-evident that no community exists in a vacuum and so every community will be influenced in some way and to some degree by its relationships with neighbours, with referral agencies, with other services, with governmental institutions, or whatever. Yet knowing this tells us relatively little about the situation of any individual community since each of these relationships is likely to vary in salience from one community to the next. In this chapter we will focus upon the different impact of the environment or operational context on therapeutic work within our communities.

In keeping with the approach adopted throughout the book we will concentrate our discussion around two communities (Faswells and Ravenscroft) and look at the remaining communities where they diverge from these two. We have chosen to concentrate on these two communities for the simple reason that much of the discussion of environmental factors in the past has crystallised around those communities operating within psychiatric hospitals. A number of writers have suggested, for example, that the hospital is an inimical host institution for therapeutic community techniques and have pointed in particular to the specialist training of doctors, the reliance on potentially unsympathetic colleagues for referrals, the hierarchical structure of the hospital, the expectations of patients, and even the medical model of illness itself, as all in some way standing at odds with the core ideas of the therapeutic community approach

(Hoffman and Singer, 1977; Manning and Blake, 1979; Myers, 1979; Reyes, 1983).

In order to assess the impact which operating within a hospital may have had on therapeutic work at Faswells and Ravenscroft we need some standard of comparison in terms of which the communities can be judged. We have chosen to concentrate here on the extensiveness of redefinitional work. By this we mean both the frequency with which redefinitional work occurred, and the range of activities in relation to which it occurred. Our reason for choosing extensiveness is simply that it is part of the core idea of the therapeutic community approach that therapy should be a continuous process across the entire range of activities occurring within the community and should be participated in by staff and residents alike. It is not surprising, then, that two of the most popular slogans associated with the approach are that 'Everything is therapy' and 'Therapy is a 24-hour process'. In the first part of this chapter we shall examine the extensiveness of the redefinitional work at Faswells and Ravenscroft and focus on the possible adverse effects of their being situated in a hospital. In the remainder of this chapter we shall look at the differences in environment of our other communities.

Faswells

Throughout the fieldwork at Faswells the question of the community's relationship to the wider hospital was very much a topical concern. There was a feeling shared by many of the Faswells staff that the relationship was at a particularly low point. Referrals to the community from other wards had dropped off; this, and the fact that the suitability for therapeutic community work of those referrals that were received was often held to be problematic, were both taken as signalling the low esteem in which Faswells was held by the hospital. 'We only get the referrals which nobody else wants' was how the Faswells consultant summed up this situation.

Similarly, amongst many of the junior nurses there was a feeling that, as a student, one had to ask specifically for a placement at Faswells since it was regarded by the nursing college tutors as an undesirable setting. In addition, Faswells staff often commented on the difficulties inherent in their relationship with the hospital administrators. We have already referred to the complaints about the filthy state of the ward from the administration, which, although accepted by Faswells staff, were nevertheless seen by them as an unwelcome intrusion into their internal domestic (in both senses of the word) affairs. At one point during the fieldwork the appointment of certain new administrative staff was seen by staff at Faswells as part of a cost-cutting exercise in which individual wards were increasingly being asked to justify themselves in cost/benefit terms. Faswells staff felt that their work could only be inadequately represented in these terms and so sought to argue their own special case. As part of this, it was somewhat reluctantly agreed by them that certain members of the administration could sit in on one of the large group meetings and see for themselves how the community operated. The large group meeting they attended, however, was full of long, empty silences and when asked by one of the residents whether they thought they might have been intruding on the work of the unit one of the visitors answered simply but devastatingly: 'I don't see anything to be intruded on here at all.' Needless to say, this comment received a good deal of heated discussion once the meeting was over and the visitors had left.

Clearly, then, in talking about Faswells' relationship with its host institution one is not talking about a relationship of peaceful co-existence. Without in any way apportioning blame to any one party, there existed something of a cold-war mentality between the community and the hospital, in which there was very little fruitful interchange between the two. However, conceding this is not the same thing as conceding that Faswells had been adversely affected by its hospital location. To make such a claim one would need to know how the community would have operated in another setting entirely. Obviously that is a question about which one can only speculate. Nevertheless, it is possible to consider the question in less general terms and look specifically at the extensiveness of redefinitional work within Faswells as compared to Ravenscroft, our other hospital-based residential community.

In Chapter 2 we described how the formal therapeutic programme in Faswells was split into a variety of large and small group meetings, art and music therapy sessions, and various other group activities. Although residents were certainly expected to 'work' on their problems in all the groups, in fact it was only the small groups and selected large groups which enjoyed anything like the regular full attendance of residents. Both the art and the music therapists operated very much on the periphery of the Faswells programme. During staff meetings, for example, a good deal of time was spent discussing the residents' work in the large groups, but only a little time was spent discussing the residents' work in the art sessions and no time at all was spent discussing their work in music therapy. One of the Faswells art therapists expressed the sense of marginality she felt in the following terms: 'I feel as if we have to regularly renegotiate our contract here, to periodically state our case and push people to get involved.' McKeganey was also well aware of how little therapeutic work appeared to occur outside the formal groups. Many of the residents associated in pairs and while there was no doubt a good deal of 'sharing' and open communication between partners, there appeared to be very little evidence of this occurring on anything like a wider informal basis. Mealtimes, for example, were very low key affairs, with most of the residents going off to eat on their own or with one or two friends. With the conclusion of the formal programme at 5.00 p.m. residents would often vacate the unit and only return late in the evening. From 9.00 p.m. there were no regular Faswells nurses on the ward but only occasional visits from one of the nurses on a different ward. At the weekends the community was virtually empty. Most of the redefinitional therapeutic work occurring in Faswells, then, was clustered around the small groups and selected large groups – those parts of the programme, that is, which were attended by the psychiatrists.

That there were marked differences in the level of involvement in redefinitional work of different staff was very evident to McKeganey early on in his fieldwork. One of the Faswells nurses commented bitterly on the paucity of therapeutic work in those meetings from which the psychiatrists were absent:

> They (the residents) will do nothing for themselves. They expect the discussion to be spoon-fed to them and will do nothing for themselves. When the doctors are there they will speak. When they're not, they don't even want to attend the meetings.

Similarly, a few weeks into the fieldwork another of the Faswells nurses asked McKeganey how the ward appeared to him:

> STAFF NURSE: You've been here a while now. Have you noticed any differences in the meetings?
>
> NM: The meetings are much quieter when the doctors are not around.
>
> STAFF NURSE: Absolutely right. When the doctors are here,

> especially the consultant, it's always much more lively.
> When they're not there are always many more silences.

To document this apparent clustering of therapeutic work around the psychiatrists McKeganey made a conscious effort to record the frequency of redefinitional work in the large groups attended only by the nurses, in those attended by the nurses *and* the psychiatrists, and in the small groups. Simplifying the results of his study somewhat, McKeganey found that interpretive redefinitions of the residents' activities were more than four times more likely to occur in those large group meetings attended by the psychiatrists than in those attended only by the nurses (McKeganey, 1986).

This clustering of redefinitional work around the psychiatrists was repeated in the small groups. Amongst both staff and residents there was a feeling that the small groups occupied a particularly important place in the therapeutic work of the unit. During the fieldwork in Faswells, for example, a number of residents were in the process of leaving the community and all, without exception, expressed a preference to continue attending their small groups on a day patient basis. To sever their connection with the small groups, then, was something residents were loath to do.

Although there was a good deal of evidence of residents participating in one another's therapy in the small groups, of asking questions, of encouraging one another to speak, and of confronting one another about things they had said or done, nevertheless the overwhelming majority of questions asked of residents, of redefinitions offered to residents, and of parallels drawn between residents, came from the psychiatrist in each group. Despite the fact that the staff membership of the groups was that of a nurse *and* a psychiatrist, the feel of the groups was very much that of a discussion orchestrated by the psychiatrists and principally involving them and the residents.

It was the psychiatrist more than either the nurses or the residents who occupied a pivotal position in the small groups. This fact was further apparent on those few occasions when the psychiatrists failed to turn up for the small groups. Instead of there being an increase in the contributions from the other members of the group – nurses and residents – at such times, there was in fact a noticeable diminution in the therapeutic work of the groups (McKeganey, 1986).

Redefinitional work in Faswells was heavily skewed in favour of certain staff roles (the psychiatrists) and certain meetings (the small groups and selected large groups). Although operating as a therapeutic community, Faswells' functioning resembled rather more closely that of the other, more traditionally run, wards elsewhere in the hospital than it did the therapeutic community ideal of therapy as a twenty-four hours a day process participated in by all staff and residents irrespective of their status.

The fact that Faswells appeared to have experienced some difficulty in operating along therapeutic community lines was something which staff themselves were well aware of and sought to explain by citing various features of their hospital location. The low numbers of referrals from colleagues, the proximity of what was regarded as an unsympathetic administration, and the expectations of residents, were all factors which staff cited as having hampered them in their work with residents.

Whilst staff certainly explained their relative lack of success in operating along therapeutic community lines in these terms, McKeganey was aware of an alternative explanation which attached rather more weight to internal social processes within Faswells. Rather than go through these in detail, which we have done elsewhere (McKeganey, 1984; McKeganey, 1986; McKeganey and Bloor, 1987), we will confine ourselves here to two salient points. First, the small groups in Faswells operated as enclaves of private communication between individual residents and individual psychiatrists from which the majority of Faswells nurses, and the art and music therapists were excluded. There was, for example, a general embargo placed upon discussing small group material outside of the small group meeting. This fact provided very favourable conditions for residents to view their communications with the psychiatrists as more important and more significant than their communications with any of the other staff. It was hardly surprising, then, to hear residents often commenting, in the company of nurses, that they preferred waiting until a 'member of staff' was present before speaking about what was bothering them. In not having access to the residents' work in the small groups most of the Faswells nurses were simply unable to engage residents on anything like an equal footing; they were, in effect, unable to break into the confidential relationships residents enjoyed with the psychiatrists, and so were unable to participate fully in the mainstream therapeutic work of the community. Second, the psychiatrists did not attend the shift change-over meetings and so the nurses coming on shift in the afternoons had no way of either continuing the work of the psychiatrists in their meetings or indeed of feeding back to the psychiatrists the sort of work which they might attempt in their meetings.

Within Faswells the apparent clustering of therapeutic work was more likely to have been the result of constraints placed upon the pooling of information amongst staff than it was the result of the community's location within a hospital setting. That Faswells staff were in effect misattributing their relative lack of success in working along therapeutic community lines to their hospital location can be seen if we look at the situation of Ravenscroft, which, since it too was operating within a hospital setting, ought also, following the logic of Faswells staff, to show signs of a comparable clustering of redefinitional work.

Ravenscroft

Like their counterparts at Faswells, staff at Ravenscroft often commented critically on their location within a hospital. There was a feeling that staff on other wards were neither particularly sympathetic to the community nor knowledgeable about its work, and that as a consequence the community often received referrals whose suitability for therapeutic community work was in doubt.

Despite these similarities in the way in which the two staff groups regarded their hospital location, however, there was very little evidence for any clustering of redefinitional work at Ravenscroft such as had occurred at Faswells. The following extract from one of the large groups demonstrates the involvement of both residents and nursing staff in the mainstream therapeutic work of the unit:

> Meeting begins at 10.00 with some chat about patients' clothes on other wards. Interrupted by Kate (resident).
>
> KATE: Do you want to say why you were feeling angry, Steve? I know you were pretty stewed up on Friday and you still seem pretty fed up.
> STEVE: My anger is not just for people in this room. I'm angry at others outside.
> GAIL (resident): Who outside?
> STEVE: I'm angry at people trying to buy my affection.
> KATE: You're angry at your mum for buying you a radio.
> STEVE: I'm angry at her for trying to buy me. I don't want to be

bought. Anyway, as far as I'm concerned it's too little too late.

SANDY (nurse): There's an interesting difference. You, Kate, were really pleased when you got that present, you just saw it for what it was.

KATE: Yes, I was just pleased that somebody thought of me.

STEVE: You can't buy love with money. It's as simple as that, it can't be got that way.

CLARE (resident): Maybe that's all she can do because you don't allow her to do anything more.

STEVE: I'm going to tell her that I don't want to see her again.

MARTIN (resident): I did that but it didn't work. That's not the way.

SANDY: The people I feel sorry for are the ones whose parents have died and who can't even talk to them. We've all got aging parents here so we know what it's like.

GAIL: I think it helps to tell your parents what you think of them. Have you told your mum how you feel about her buying you the radio?

STEVE: No.

GAIL: I saw my mum at the weekend in London. It had been arranged but I didn't really want to go. She started buying me things, cigs and things and I hated her for it, for all of the things she hasn't given me or what I feel she hasn't given me. And I told her. I know it hurt her, I could see it, but it made me feel a lot better that I had spoken about it and it made me feel that I didn't hate her so much.

SANDY: I think we all have a nice little fantasy that if we ever tell our parents what we really feel about them they would die on the spot. The reality of course is very different.

STEVE: Maybe I'll write to my mum and say we should have a chat. I'm not interested in speaking to the old man because he knows what I think of *him*.

SANDY: O.K. I think we're going to have to close it there.

Although there were no clinical staff present at this meeting, residents showed no less an inclination to question or confront each other. Equally, Sandy, the nurse, was quite prepared to interpret residents' behaviour and to draw parallels between residents. The fact that the psychiatrists were absent from the group was, quite simply, an irrelevancy in terms of the therapeutic content of the meeting.

Redefinitional work was also very evident in the small groups, though without any of the clustering that was apparent in Faswells. In fact, the Ravenscroft consultant did not even attend the small groups which were run by the psychologist and the art therapist. Although to avoid overloading the small groups not all of the Ravenscroft nurses were able to attend the meetings, nevertheless staff placed a good deal of emphasis on pooling the contents of residents' work in the small groups amongst the entire staff group and would hold regular meetings to achieve this end. In this way even those staff members who were unable to attend the groups were still kept abreast of the residents' work in the small groups and were able to raise items of small group discussion at other points in the formal programme.

In contrast to the situation at Faswells, redefinitional therapeutic work was spread throughout the Ravenscroft programme and occurred not only in the large and small groups but also in the art therapy sessions. Also, a good deal of time was spent discussing the art work in the staff meetings. As we noted in Chapter 3, a portfolio of each resident's art work was kept in the staff room and used for the periodic art therapy reviews, during which recurring images in the residents' paintings would be explored with the art therapist. Staff coming on shift after a period of absence were often seen leafing through these portfolios as a way of updating their knowledge of individual residents. Evening shift change-over meetings and emergency large group meetings called by residents were also important arenas for staff and resident redefinitional work:

> Evening hand-over. David (staff nurse) complains that Elinor (resident), having been unable to get on a bus to attend her evening class, returned in a state requesting an audience with Kathy (nurse). David says Elinor should have called a meeting 'since this way all that happens is that the rest of the community feels excluded'. Elinor looks resentful but ten minutes after the hand-over the house bell announcing an emergency meeting is rung by Carol, Elinor's close friend. Carol explains her feelings of despair and of wanting to kill herself: 'I can't hold myself together any longer, I feel as if I'm coming apart.' Everyone including me is waiting to hear what Elinor is going to say. She answers that there is nothing to be said. David (staff nurse) says there is and goes on to criticise Elinor for not calling the meeting, repeating his earlier point about excluding the group. Elinor then

> describes her feelings of anxiety at the bus stop. Richard (resident) suggests that by psyching herself up for the class she is creating another failure for herself. Carol agrees and says Elinor is trying to do too much too soon. The other residents chip in similar views and it is finally agreed that Elinor should drop the class. Though I personally think it might be better for her to continue, I'm really impressed at how much concern the other residents have shown Elinor.

Despite similarities in their resident populations, in their approach to therapy, and in their hospital location, there were striking differences between these two communities in the extensiveness of redefinitional work. At Faswells such work appeared to be clustered around the psychiatrists and restricted largely to selected large groups and the small groups. At Ravenscroft it was distributed throughout both the formal and informal programme and involved all of the staff and residents. Although Faswells staff explained their own difficulties in operationalising a model of therapeutic community practice by citing their location within a hospital setting, the fact that Ravenscroft staff did not appear to have experienced comparable difficulties suggests that it was not the hospital location itself which had influenced redefinitional work at Faswells but some factors internal to that community which were not shared by Ravenscroft. We have suggested that the limited pooling of information amongst staff at Faswells may well have been the root cause of the contraction of therapeutic work in that community relative to Ravenscroft, where there was a good deal of pooling of information on all aspects of the residents' work.

Whilst it is undoubtedly the case that therapeutic communities may be adversely affected by their placement within a hospital setting, the contrasting experiences of Faswells and Ravenscroft suggest that that influence is neither inevitable nor unavoidable. In the remainder of this chapter we shall concentrate upon the role of the environment for each of our other communities.

The other communities

Although staff at both Faswells and Ravenscroft differed in the extent to which they saw themselves as having been hampered by working within a hospital setting they did at least agree in that they saw nothing about their environment which in any way assisted their work with residents. The situation of Parkneuk in this respect was very different.

Partly because of the rural location of Parkneuk, and partly because of their very different approach to therapy, staff sought to make active, therapeutic use of parts of their environment – most notably their relationships with neighbours. Staff encouraged residents to attend local community events and even sought to place the more capable residents in local jobs. The foster-familial therapeutic approach within Parkneuk extended outside the community as staff sought to maintain open, friendly and reciprocal relationships with various neighbours.

> With a few of the locals relationships are very good, especially the McBride family. Mrs McBride, local postmistress, is on the Parkneuk council of trustees and used to allow Philip (resident) to come in and watch her television. Mr McBride is a local farmworker who has done various good turns for the community.

Parkneuk's integration into the local community was further facilitated by having one of the staff members sit on the local village hall committee. In this way the community was kept abreast of any forthcoming local events and residents were easily able to make an input into these. Staff benefited from these reciprocal relationships in two obvious ways. First, they were released from having to provide a programme of leisure activities for residents – something which they had tried to do in the past and found very difficult to organise. Second, through their contacts with local families, residents were gradually socialised into the skills and reality of communal living which would equip them in any move on to a village-type setting like Newton Dee.

Whilst the community undoubtedly enjoyed a positive relationship with neighbouring families, staff recognised the potential fragility of these relationships and were very conscious of the need not to appear odd or strange in the eyes of neighbouring families:

> We are rolling a bean bed. The roller is a tree-trunk attached to a wooden frame and pulled by two people with chains. Mark (staff) comments 'It's a good job the local farmworkers can't see us now'.

Similarly on another occasion:

> In the afternoon everyone comes out to roll and tramp the rye grass. I suggest we join hands to ensure that we keep together but Mark doesn't like the idea because he doesn't want us to be noticed by the neighbours.

Despite this fragility, relationships with neighbours were on the whole very positive. Relationships with residents' parents, on the other hand, were more problematic. Staff regarded the parents' annual visits as little more than inhibiting distractions and would often comment unfavourably on the parents' unrealistic wishes and plans for their son or daughter. However, since these visits only usually occurred once a year, parents were not really able to influence the therapeutic work to any noticeable degree.

Referrals to Parkneuk were routed through the Camphill medical consultant and while staff were not entirely in agreement with what they saw as the consultant's preference for referring disturbed adolescents to them, this had not surfaced to anything like the extent that it had at Faswells. This is not of course to suggest that the relationships between Parkneuk and referral agencies were all sweetness and light. In Chapter 4 we mentioned the disagreement between staff and one particular resident's social worker as to whether the resident in question ought to focus her attention on her new relationships in the house (as staff believed), or on her relationship with her parents (as her social worker believed). Parkneuk staff, however, were able to smooth over the disagreement, continue their work with the resident, and maintain their relationship with the social worker in question.

Despite their many similarities, Parkneuk and Camphill were very different as far as relationships with the external environment were concerned. Whereas Parkneuk staff sought to maximise the interaction between the community and its neighbours, the aim at Camphill was much more one of creating a rather closed environment around the children in which Steiner's principles of communal living and curative work could be applied. This is not, of course, to suggest that the relationship between Camphill and its surrounding community was entirely neglected. There was, for example, a local 'Friends of Camphill' committee which would fund-raise and support the community in various ways. Nevertheless, Camphill was much more self-supportive than Parkneuk, more

Utopian in its vision and, as a consequence, more self-enclosed in its work. This fact was often most apparent when co-workers took the children on trips outside the community and confronted the very different views of the children held by some of the local shopkeepers:

> This afternoon I accompanied Kirsten and Hans (co-workers) on a trip outside the community. On the way to the bus some of the children wanted to buy sweets and things in the local shop. It was Saturday afternoon and I suppose the staff were pretty harassed but I could tell on top of this a certain wariness both on their part and that of the co-workers as the children wandered around the shop. It was impossible to keep an eye on them all but that was clearly what the assistants were trying to do. As we left I asked Kirsten why the staff seemed so unfriendly. She explained that it was because they had no understanding of the children's inquisitiveness and thought that they were all the time looking to steal things.

While Camphill differed from Parkneuk as far as their relationships with neighbours were concerned, the two communities were rather similar in their view of parents. Although Camphill staff regarded it as very important that the children return to their own homes at various points throughout the year, they viewed the visits of parents to the community as something of a disruptive influence. Staff would often point out, for example, that in the period surrounding these visits the children would be more disturbed than usual and would need time to settle down. However, the fact that many of the parents would have had to travel long distances, coupled with the fact that staff did not encourage regular visits, meant that parents were again poorly placed to have any influence on the therapeutic work of the community.

As far as relationships with the children's social workers were concerned, the situation was different again. Although many of the children did have an appointed social worker it was only very infrequently that they visited the community. When they did, however, they would receive VIP treatment, with staff making special efforts to describe the details of the community's work to them and the nature of the individual child's progress. In part, of course, this is hardly surprising, since the continued financial support of the child's local authority would depend at least in part on the reports social workers provided of the Camphill placement.

Despite Camphill's attempts to separate itself from its surrounding environment, it is undoubtedly the case that no community can be entirely uninfluenced by its environment. The publication of the Warnock Report (1978), proposing the incorporation of mentally handicapped children into the community as opposed to their placement within special schools, could have signalled a death-knell for settings like Camphill. In fact, Camphill was able to argue a case for itself which has ensured its continued survival in spite of this shift in policy. Nevertheless, Camphill's experience in this respect does illustrate just how influential environmental factors can be in determining not only what happens *within* communities, but also the potential fate of communities themselves.

On the whole the concept house enjoyed fairly positive relationships with its surrounding environment, most notably with the intake/detoxification unit from which referrals were received and the halfway house to which discharges were made.

In a way that was rather reminiscent of Faswells, the administrator of the concept house, however, was very keen to establish objective outcome criteria in order to compare the effectiveness of the concept house against other similar facilities in the area, such as a methadone programme. Concept house staff, though, were critical of such a move and were sceptical of the feasibility of producing such criteria in the first place, given the complex nature of their work. While staff were able to resist such an evaluation they were not able to resist the climate of financial restraint placed upon the health and personal social services generally. As a result of pressure to reduce their costs the expected length of stay of residents in the Dutch concept houses had been reduced from one year to six months.

The situation at the day hospital was somewhat similar to that at Faswells and Ravenscroft since staff repeatedly complained about the paucity of referrals from colleagues on other wards. Indeed, as we stated in Chapter 2, patient numbers in the day hospital dropped to as low as eight at one point during the fieldwork.

It would be absurd to suggest that this fact had not influenced therapeutic work at all in the unit. One very obvious way in which low numbers had influenced activities occurring within the community was in the need to avoid overloading the groups with staff members. The strategy of having patients express their preference for the staff composition of the group was adopted as one way of avoiding this overloading. However, it would be wrong to suggest that low numbers had necessarily led to a diminution in the therapeutic work of the unit, at least as far as those patients who were attending the day hospital were concerned. In fact, a good deal of redefinitional material was produced precisely from having patients express their preference for staff membership of the groups.

Although the external environment of the day hospital had undoubtedly had some impact on therapeutic work in the unit, there was none of the clustering of redefinitional work around certain staff roles and certain parts of the programme that was evident at Faswells. Once again, we must conclude that the simple fact of operating within a hospital does not in itself mean that one will be unable to employ therapeutic community treatment techniques, even if it does influence the context within which those techniques are employed.

We turn finally to Ashley and Beeches. Since both of these communities were similarly circumstanced, with the same parent organisation, and similar client groups, we shall discuss them together.

It is probably true to say that residential work with maladjusted or disturbed adolescents is the one arrangement most likely to give rise to difficulties with neighbours in the surrounding community. Certainly staff in both houses were well aware of this and on occasion at least would take steps to prevent conflicts arising or resolve them once they had arisen. The warden at Ashley, for example, commented to Bloor that he had put a lot of work into maintaining friendly relationships with neighbours and instanced how he recently had to deal with a complaint from a neighbour at having her doorbell rung by some of the residents. While staff did not greatly enjoy smoothing over such problems they did recognise the importance of not antagonising or alienating the local community. As it happens, staff in both houses had been able to foster fairly positive contacts with their local communities. During his fieldwork in Beeches, for example, Bloor attended a house party at which members of the 'Friends of Beeches' committee were also present:

> Many of the guests at the party were members of the Friends of Beeches, a body of local supporters and fund-raisers (among them the GP, the next-door neighbours, and a probation officer). Earlier that day they had provided a table tennis table. They mixed with the residents with informality – dancing, playing games, even playing darts in a side room. Staff had ensured that many had been invited by particular residents and residents were

> encouraged to look after their guests; when one couple left Sally (staff) told Tom (resident) to show his guests to the door and say goodbye.

Although this managed sociability was one way of maintaining positive relationships with the local community it was also of benefit in instructing residents in the sorts of social skills necessary for their future independent living.

Relationships with other agencies in the area were rather more problematic, and in both houses there was further evidence of this managed sociability on the part of staff. Relationships with the police were a good example of this:

> The community police constable dropped by for coffee at coffee time. Danny's (resident) disappearance was discussed and the PC said he'd keep an eye open for him. Doreen (resident) let slip that he'd been nicking things in the house and later Carol (staff) ticked her off for letting that out in front of him. Doreen admitted that she had done it on purpose because she was so brassed off with Danny. Carol asked her how she would like it if people informed on *her* to the police.

Similarly, on another occasion, the warden at Ashley commented that the reason staff were on fairly good terms with the local police was because they had never attempted to argue with them.

Although staff in both houses felt that they had a fairly good working relationship with referral agencies, they were well aware of the need to maintain a clear view of their own needs and capabilities relative to those of staff in other agencies:

> Staff meeting: Talking about possible new residents, Mark (warden) contrasted two referrals: one concerned a transsexual who needed a place to experiment with becoming a woman before undergoing a sex-change operation; another concerned a girl made homeless by the closure of a local halfway house. Mark said social workers couldn't both expect the house to be a shelter for emergency cases and a place for helping someone through a massive identity change; the two weren't compatible.

Likewise, staff commented that there were occasions when referring local authorities would attempt to 'dump' their most difficult adolescents on them:

> Caroline (staff) talking about relationships with social services departments: generally good relationships now with departments who have a good idea of what would be an appropriate referral and what the house does. Mark (warden) had previously remarked that some departments view them with awe as having taken on and transformed children with long histories of residential care who had been perpetual thorns in the side of their social workers. Occasionally departments have tried to dump kids here to the extent of failing to inform the house about histories of arson and the like. Some sad tales about cases who have made a lot of progress here but then may falter after leaving.

Finally, there was some evidence that staff in both houses felt themselves to be constrained in their work with residents by their relationships with the parent organisation. Some of the staff were sceptical, for example, of what they took to be the rather academic approach of headquarters staff, while others commented unfavourably on what they saw as the increasing amounts of administrative work they were being called upon to do:

> Martine (staff) proudly showed me last year's returns which indicated that the house had achieved the highest earnings of any of the existing adolescent houses. Mentioned her irritation with the increasing amounts of administration work demanded of house staff by HQ. She instanced how she now had to file details of every journey on house business outside the house. Complained that this work took staff away from their therapeutic work.

Within both Ashley and Beeches, then, there was some evidence of various aspects of the environment operating as a constraining factor on staff work.

Summary and conclusion

In this chapter we have attempted to explore the impact of the environment, or operational context, on activities taking place within our communities. We concentrated on Faswells and Ravenscroft for the simple reason that the strongest case for the environment of the community having a decisive impact on work within therapeutic communities has been made in relation to those communities operating within or alongside hospitals. Hospitals, it has been suggested, are among the least favourable environments for the implementation of therapeutic community techniques.

Our study has only partially borne this out. Although staff at Faswells, Ravenscroft and the day hospital all commented unfavourably about some aspects of their hospital location, it was only at Faswells that staff explained their difficulties in operating along therapeutic community lines by citing aspects of their location – most notably the proximity of unsympathetic colleagues and administrators, and the expectations of residents on entering a hospital. However, the fact that it was only in Faswells that there was a noticeable clustering of redefinitional work around certain staff roles and certain parts of the programme suggests that this may have had rather less to do with Faswells' hospital location per se than with social processes within Faswells which were not shared by our other hospital-based communities. In particular we suggested that the position of the small groups as enclaves of confidential communication between psychiatrists and residents, along with the very limited pooling of information generally, may have been at the root of the clustering of redefinitional work evident in Faswells.

As far as our remaining communities are concerned we have sought to show the enormous variability both in the constituents of the different environments, and in the influence they are seen to exert. Whilst we would accept the general idea that therapeutic communities may be influenced by having to operate within certain contexts we would regard it as an oversimplification to suggest that that influence is always entirely negative. We described the situation of Parkneuk, for example, where, although staff were constrained in some ways by the nearness of neighbours, nevertheless in other ways they sought to make active use of neighbours by including them in the mainstream therapeutic work of the community.

Similarly, we would reject the suggestion that environmental factors exert an unavoidable influence on therapeutic community work. The situation of the day hospital is particularly interesting in this respect since staff there had actively sought to make themselves more accessible to staff on other wards as one way of overcoming what they saw as some of the difficulties of having to operate within a hospital setting, for example, having to depend for referrals on colleagues who were either antagonistic to the day hospital's approach or insufficiently knowledgeable about the treatment methods:

> Michael (staff) brought me up to date with staff discussions yesterday about the continuing low patient numbers and the worries about this if it were to continue (one possibility would be reductions in staff because of staff shortages elsewhere in the hospital). Staff had decided that they would perhaps have to change the format of the day hospital, that they'd been 'too rigid' (or seen to be too rigid), that they ought to consider running different sorts of groups for different sorts of patients with different levels of intensity. Michael talked about having one-day-a-week groups for those who couldn't leave their work, marital therapy groups instead of individual marital therapy. He also said they should consider the possibility of catering for a wider spread of disabilities and being more flexible in their assessments of new patients (including making referral easier for referring psychiatrists by making it clear that they were prepared to consider patients on days other than Monday).

While we are not suggesting that therapeutic community practitioners can solve all of their difficulties of working in unfavourable environments simply by adopting the techniques of impression management (Goffman, 1959), we do feel that the situation of some communities could be enhanced by adopting a more flexible stance – not, we should add, by sacrificing the underlying principles of their work, but rather by looking for ways to make their work more accessible to others.

This chapter concludes our discussion of substantive topics in relation to our communities. In the following chapter we will aim to conclude the book by concentrating on, among other things, the common properties of redefinitional work shared across our communities.

Chapter 7
Conclusions

In Hilaire Belloc's book *Path to Rome* there is a section entitled 'In Praise of this Book'. His example has not been widely followed: authors are generally somewhat coy and circumspect in drawing the reader's attention to the worth and uses of their books. We shall follow tradition in this respect but depart from it in another: we have chosen to represent the implications of our work separately for the different audiences – therapeutic community practitioners, sociologists, and general readers – who might have an interest in this study. We are not trying to hedge our bets, nor are we trying to stipulate who can have an interest in what, but rather we want to give explicit recognition to the fact that different audiences will lay different emphases on different aspects of the same findings. If implications lie in the eye of the beholder, the researchers should take this into account in the presentation of their conclusions.

For a practitioner audience, we have listed particular practices found in just one or two communities in our sample, practices which are highlighted by a comparative perspective and which appear to promote therapy in the settings where they are found. Since many practitioners lack a detailed knowledge of more than two or three contrasting approaches to therapeutic community treatment, we hope that by furnishing this list we shall provide a stimulus to experiment and cross-fertilisation. We do not suggest that the practices on our list are suitable for blanket application, but all of them could be adopted more widely than they are at present.

For a sociological audience, we have tried to draw out what has hitherto been largely implicit in our analysis, namely the central properties found in all therapeutic community work. These central properties are differentially extensible and so comprise a conceptual framework for representing variations in practice across different settings. We compare our own approach with other sociological conceptions of therapeutic work in order to assess the utility of this approach for sociological studies of therapeutic work in other areas of medical practice.

For a general readership, we draw on aspects of our earlier discussion (volition and therapy, power and resistance) to assess the potential of therapeutic communities as agencies of social change. We suggest that some types of communities may offer a remedy for what Ivan Illich, arch-critic of professional medicine, has called 'structural iatrogenesis' – the expropriation of the power of individuals and collectivities to heal themselves (Illich, 1975).

Implications for therapeutic community practitioners

Our study has been descriptive rather than 'evaluative' in the conventional sense. This is not a matter for apology, since we do not believe that the conventional evaluative research design (derived from trials of pharmacological treatments) is appropriate for evaluating complex organisations and non-standardised treatments (see our methods appendix). However, because of the equation of evaluation with these conventional experimental research designs, it is easy to lose sight of the fact that any comparative description of treatment agencies is in fact implicitly 'evaluative' in the broad sense of the term. Comparative description juxtaposes similar and contrasting practices in such a manner as to facilitate evaluative judgments by both researchers and readers.

At some points in our study the evaluative relevance of our comparative descriptions will have been perfectly obvious, as in our linking of inadequate communications between psychiatrists and nurses at Faswells to the erosion of the community programme (see Chapter 6). At other points evaluative relevance has remained implicit and unstated, a matter of silent judgment by the researchers. We take the opportunity to remedy that here. We shall concentrate in this section on drawing out this implicit evaluative relevance, pointing out some aspects of practice highlighted by our comparisons which *may* be associated with effective practice – with reduced defaulting rates, with the promotion of resident reflectivity, with combatting resident institutionalisation, and so on. We emphasise that these particular practices 'may' be associated with effectiveness: we cannot claim a definite relationship, for such a claim would demand controlled studies which are notoriously difficult to mount. Nor would we claim that our 'list' of particular practices is exhaustive; we simply refer to those aspects of practice in individual communities which have struck us as promoting effectiveness in the course of our analysis. And one final disclaimer: we realise that these aspects of practice, presently unique to one or two communities, may not always be capable of straightforward transfer to other settings; they may clash with other valued practices, they may require additional inputs of staff or resources, they may involve unacceptable rescheduling of timetables, and so on.

We have chosen to list seven aspects of practice, presently found in only one or two communities in our sample, but capable in principle of extension to some at least of the other communities we have described. We could have presented more than seven practices but we feel that the additions would lack the relevance of our present list. We present them in no particular or hierarchical order.

1 Making fellow residents responsible for keeping residents in treatment

None of the communities we studied were custodial institutions, and so all of them were to some extent vulnerable to premature departures by residents. As in any course of treatment, those who discontinue treatment prematurely can be expected to derive less benefit than those who remain for the full course. In some types of therapeutic community, notably the concept houses, the high proportion of defaulters has led critics to question the efficacy of the treatment, despite good results from follow-up studies among those who complete treatment.

No community is more vulnerable to defaulting than a day hospital, where defaulting is simply a matter of going home at the end of one day and failing to return to the hospital on the next day. At the Ross Clinic day hospital a practice had evolved which met this difficulty: fellow patients were made largely responsible for keeping patients in treatment. Patients who ran out of groups in tears were likely to be followed by one or more of their fellows to comfort them and ensure their return. Patients thought to be under particular strain were sometimes sought out by their fellows with offers of company in the evenings and at weekends. And patients who failed to turn up at the hospital could expect a deputation of fellow-patients (sometimes with a staff-member) to visit them at home and attempt to persuade them to return to the hospital, unless they had formally announced and discussed their intentions to leave in one of the community groups.

This practice was not without its drawbacks. The provision of comfort and support for distressed patients could be seen by staff as buttressing patients' resistance to talking about their problems in the groups. Again, mutual support among patients could sometimes be seen as 'splitting': the formation of exclusive pair-bonds and cliques. And further, some patients who stayed away from the hospital were thought to be aware that they would be chased after and visited; this might be characterised as attention-seeking. It may be responded that none of these drawbacks was in fact crucial since all these points could be raised by staff and dealt with in the course of the groups; in our terminology they could become occasions and topics of redefinitional work.

The value of the practice was threefold. First, it reduced defaulting; second, it extended patients' involvement in one another's therapy; and third, by making patients primarily responsible for maintaining their fellows in treatment, it eased staff inhibitions about placing patients (some of whom were para-suicides) under pressure in the course of group treatment.

Some of the residential communities could, in principle, adopt this day hospital practice of maintaining potential defaulters in treatment. At Ashley, for example, residents were already accustomed to welcoming new arrivals and offering them support to overcome their sense of estrangement and/or homesickness. However, Ashley residents who were assimilated into the peer group, and who resolved to default, were not prevented by their fellow-residents, who made peer group loyalties paramount. Recall the defaulting resident mentioned in Chapter 5 who intercepted the postman to secure his giro order (welfare benefit): a number of residents were aware of his intentions but did nothing to dissuade him, and one fellow-resident in fact helped the defaulter carry his bags to the bus station.

2 *The institutionalised aftergroup for the promotion of reflectivity*

In a number of communities the 'highlight' of the group programme is the weekly 'community meeting'. This is especially the case in halfway houses where many residents are absent from the house, and the group programme, during the day. Issues relating to the government and governance of the community are discussed, but it is also seen as a forum for the discussion of continuing difficulties, residents' plans for the future, and inter-personal disputes. Emotions often run high: tears, screamed abuse, laughter and hugging are frequent occurrences.

Staff are well aware that the aftermath of these emotional outbursts represents a potential problem of management. At Beeches halfway house, for example, it was the practice to split the meeting into two sections – a prior, open, and flexible section to give free rein to the expression of feelings, followed by a highly ordered business section. The rationale for this division and sequencing was that the low-key, efficient conduct of the business section gave residents a structured opportunity to wind down after the emotional maelstrom of the earlier part of the meeting.

At Ashley halfway house a different procedure was in operation which similarly gave residents the opportunity to wind down, but had wider potential benefits insofar as it provided a structured opportunity for residents to describe and reflect on their feelings and behaviour. We are referring to the half-hour 'aftergroup'. Immediately following the community meeting, and prior to the staff meeting, staff and residents would leave the large living room where the community meeting had been held and adjourn to the kitchen and the adjoining dining room. Someone would put on the kettle for coffee and the biscuits would be unearthed from their hiding place in the staff flat. Once the kettle had boiled, someone would bellow out 'Aftergroup!' to alert late-comers. Without further ado, nearly everyone (attendance was optional) would sit down around the dining-room table with their coffee and biscuits and discuss, joke, and reminisce about the events of the community meeting and how they had felt about it:

> Maggie (resident), who had done a lot of work in the [community meeting], spoke about having the shakes during [the meeting] and how it had been the first time she'd ever lost her temper and shouted in a group; she spoke a lot in the aftergroup and gradually returned to joking and normality.

As we stressed in Chapter 3, reality-confronting communities seek to make residents observers of their own behaviour and associated feeling-states. Reflecting on, and expressing, feelings are in fact *learned* activities. The half-hour aftergroup, following hard on the heels of the tumultuous emotional events of the community group, offered an occasion for residents to develop (with encouragement and example from others) a practised ability to reflect on their feelings and actions.

Some of the reality-confronting communities in our sample already possessed similar organisational devices to promote such reflectivity. At the day hospital, for example, groups were scheduled to follow immediately on from the twice-weekly activity groups and the weekly encounter group, so that patients' behaviour in those preceding groups could be a topic for discussion. We are merely suggesting the adoption of the aftergroup mechanism in settings where no approximation currently exists.

3 *The attendance of residents at staff change-over meetings*

Some of our communities (for example, Camphill) did not operate a staff shift system, but all those that did operate with shift-working made use of staff change-over meetings for out-going staff to acquaint in-coming staff with the latest developments in the community. In two of our communities, Ravenscroft and Ashley, residents were allowed (but not required) to attend these change-over meetings.

There was thought to be some value in resident attendance insofar as it defused residents' suspicions about what went on at these meetings; in the terminology we adopted in Chapter 5, dominance was reduced when the therapeutic gaze was no longer disembodied, no longer a collective construct framed behind closed doors. But the main value of the residents' attendance was seen to lie in the further opportunity it presented for residents to hear their behaviour described by the out-going staff, to see themselves through the eyes of others. Recall our description in Chapter 3 of the residents' sense of self as a social being as a 'looking glass self' (Cooley, 1983): residents' attendance at change-over meetings in reality-confronting communities simply provides a further opportunity for staff to hold their mirror up to residents and confront them with the picture of their behaviour as seen by others, a further opportunity for residents to come to see their own behaviour as inappropriate and unacceptable.

We are aware that the logic of the position outlined here would lead to allowing residents access to all settings (staff review groups, files and reports) where residents are discussed. Indeed, the question of such access has been debated in some communities. But we recognise that there are difficulties in the extension of resident access, not least because it would allow a resident's peers access to information about that resident which the resident might wish to remain confidential within the staff group. It might thus be judged less controversial if the extension of residential access were confined to the change-over meetings, where the topics of discussion are likely to be the immediate past of which all in the community have knowledge. Note, however, that some communities in our sample (Ashley and Parkneuk) allowed the resident concerned access to the staff reports to the resident's referral agency, and Ashley residents also had the opportunity of recording a dissenting opinion at the end of the report if they so wished.

4 The 'tight house' as a device to counteract institutionalisation

Sharp (1975) has written at length about the 'neo-institutionalisation' of residents in a therapeutic community, and it is certain that instrumental communities in particular (because of the relatively lengthy careers of their residents) face a potential problem of institutionalised resident adaptation to the community regime. A common organisational device in concept houses to combat institutionalisation is the periodic 'tight house'. In the tight house, the house director and his/her assistants take over the everyday running of the house, senior residents lose their positions in the status hierarchy and these are made open to competition from all residents, 'therapeutic measures' are increased, privileges such as phone calls are suspended, and poorly motivated residents are assigned to the 'prospect chair' reserved for new arrivals (to be allowed to stay they must demonstrate their commitment and take a 'shaved head').

It may be that the 'tight house' is the organised and orchestrated equivalent of the 'oscillations' that Rapoport (1960, p. 167) noted in his study of the reality-confronting community at Henderson Hospital, which he in turn tied to the periodic 'collective upsets' which seem to be a natural phenomenon in all psychiatric institutions. If this is the case, then it may be desirable for all communities to attempt to adopt tailor-made equivalents of the 'tight house' to be applied deliberately and periodically to combat institutionalisation on the part of both staff and residents. Instrumental communities with a status hierarchy might be able to adopt a tight house programme similar to that of the concept houses. Reality-confronting communities would have to adopt different strategies, say, the cancellation of the programme in favour of open-ended community meetings, the commissioning of small groups to report back on solutions to identified problems, and so on. The advantage of the tight house device lies, of course, in the planned anticipation of crises rather than extemporary reaction to them.

We recognise that not all crises can be so anticipated: for example, crises can be precipitated by external factors beyond the ken and control of the community, although our research leads us to suspect that the deleterious impact of external events on therapeutic work may be less than is commonly claimed (see Chapter 6). Even so, the individually tailored equivalent of the tight house provides a ready-made organisational framework through which the community may respond.

5 *Devices for increasing resident awareness of the mutability of community structure*

Staff who have seen many changes in the organisational structure of their community are sometimes shocked to discover that residents, from their shorter temporal perspective, may regard that structure as fixed and immutable. This apparent misperception by residents has consequences for the therapeutic work of the community. With the exception of the concept houses, all communities, be they reality-confronting or instrumental, are formally democratic, with the government and governance of the community open in principle to debate and modification. This is not to say that the communities are wholly democratic: democracy is one of the creative 'myths' of therapeutic community practice (Morrice, 1972). In participating in the community's democratic forms, in encountering and disputing the limits to democracy, residents both reveal their difficulties to the therapeutic gaze of the staff and have the opportunity to learn to adapt to thwarted expectations in non-pathogenic ways. In learning to accept the defeasible character of therapeutic community democracy, residents may come to accept the defeasible character of expectations and behavioural prescriptions in everyday life (Bloor and Fonkert, 1982). By contrast, a perception by residents of the structure of the community as immutable, or the government of the community as the preserve of the senior staff, lessens the participation by residents in government and organisational change, and without that participation opportunities for therapy are lost. Our research has given us acquaintanceship with two devices that may increase resident awareness of the mutability of the community structure: a collective visit to a second community where the organisation is different, and the Beeches 'Think Day'.

The visit of Faswells residents and staff to a second community during the period of McKeganey's fieldwork led to comparisons being drawn between the two communities, and led Faswells residents to discuss the possibility of certain changes in structure and practice at their community. For example, meals at Faswells were delivered from the hospital kitchens and residents would simply collect their meals individually and taken them away to eat in private. Following the visit, there was a considerable discussion about the possibility of making the mealtimes a community occasion, as they had been at the second community. The participation of residents in such discussions, regardless of the eventual outcome of those discussions, provides an occasion for therapeutic work – for monitoring residents' behaviour, for pointing out inappropriate behaviour, for trying out new patterns of behaviour, and so on. The Association of Therapeutic Communities, to which many communities are affiliated, is a forum for cross-fertilisation among members and has provided a stimulus for such inter-community visits. We hope this book may also stimulate interest in such visits.

In instrumental communities with a formally democratic structure, such as Beeches, participation in democratic discussion was valued, not as an occasion for reality-confrontation, but as evidence of resident acceptance of the new social reality of the community, and as a channel for funnelling resident grievances into legitimate rather than subcultural channels. If residents perceive the community to be recalcitrant to democratic change, then the effectiveness of the instrumental regime is naturally reduced – 'secondary adjustments' (Goffman, 1968) – and deviant subcultures would be probable consequences.

The Beeches 'Think Day' was a neat rebuttal of the charge of oligarchy and a practical demonstration of the mutability of the community structure. The first 'Think Day' was held during Bloor's fieldwork; it was planned to hold further ones periodically at the warden's discretion. The event began with the elicitation of topics from residents that they would like to discuss ('I didn't realise you were so happy with the house rules, Terry?'). A long list was quickly contributed, including some staff suggestions: topics ranged from the suggested abolition of the 'no violence' rule to the setting up of a house darkroom for photographers. Members were asked to divide themselves into groups of four with a minute-taker and a chairman; staff ensured that no group was composed wholly of residents.

Each group chose its own topics and was asked to discuss each in turn and then report back to the meeting. For example, Bloor's group had as one of its four topics the house 'no violence' rule. Lenny, who had suggested the topic, urged that people who got into fights should just be left to themselves – staff should not intervene. The staff role, in the warden's view, was that of guide rather than disputant. So Bloor asked what his fellow group members thought would happen if fights were allowed to take their course: Would there be more bullying? Would there be more damage to the property? The group unanimously agreed to recommend no change in the rule.

Nevertheless, some changes were recommended and adopted. For example, it was recommended and adopted that residents should no longer be put on house restriction if they returned to the house in the evenings within fifteen minutes of the appointed time: they should simply forfeit the amount they had exceeded their curfew on a subsequent night. Again, it was recommended and adopted that residents who performed satisfactorily during the day's programme should have the privilege of an extra half-hour before their bedtimes. Proposals about which the warden was unenthusiastic could be deferred by the device of claiming that the house's headquarters organisation would need to approve the change or agree the necessary expenditure – a proposal for a residents' 'private room' (no staff access without invitation) fell into this category.

By their very participation in the exercise residents were led to subscribe to the democratic ethos of the house, to the legitimacy of the house structure, and to the consensual and mutable character of the house rules. Of course, we do not suggest that the Think Day ensured that Beeches was an unequivocally democratic regime: there were limits to democracy – witness the residents' 'private room' issue. Rather, the Think Day exercise helped to *construct* the Beeches regime as a democracy in the eyes of the residents, and similar exercises – we suggest – might give similar results in other communities.

6 *Resident selection of participating staff*

Reference has already been made in passing to the day hospital practice of requiring patients to express preferences about which staff they wanted in the groups during periods when patient numbers were low (see Chapter 4). In the large group on Monday mornings staff would state whether or not they would be available to work in the groups that week, and patients would be asked to choose, from those available, the staff members that they would prefer to work with that week.

When the practice began, its avowed purpose was to prevent staff over-weighting of the groups at a time when patient numbers were low. However, in the course of its operation staff discovered these patient choices provided an occasion and a topic for therapeutic work. Staff over-weighting was seen as a problem, not just because it was an inefficient use of staff resources, but also because it reduced the extent of reality-confrontation by fellow-patients, and such peer-group confrontations were thought to be more effective than those conducted by staff. The therapeutic work associated with patient choices centred on the reasons that might be adduced and inferred for particular patients' preferences for, and antipathies toward, particular members of staff, but discussions could also be heard on how patients' choices reflected irresponsibility or manipulative intent. It seems likely that if certain members of staff were persistently included or excluded on the basis of patients' choices then this would occasion discussions about performance within the staff team, but Bloor's fieldwork at the day hospital only encompassed one period of low patient numbers wherein patient choices were exercised.

Many communities are likely to suffer from occasional down-turns in resident numbers. This is particularly the case in communities with short resident careers, where stability of numbers depends either on regularity in referrals or the operation of a waiting list for admission. There is also the suggestion that hospital-based communities are experiencing a long-term down-turn in referral numbers, associated with an increasing preference among psychiatrists for organic treatments (administered on an out-patient basis) in respect of those types of patient disorder from which hospital communities have traditionally drawn their patients.

The two remaining hospital-based communities in our sample (Ravenscroft and Faswells) both reported periodic problems in securing adequate referrals. Under these circumstances, it seems possible that the day hospital practice reported here could be more widely adopted.

However, it may be that the apparent therapeutic advantages of resident selection of participating staff would recommend the adoption of the practice even where there were no difficulties with resident numbers. For example, residents might be asked periodically to choose the staff member(s) with whom they preferred to work in work groups or in their small groups. Such periodic resident choices of staff might be combined with staff rotation between small groups to avoid 'splitting'. We advance these suggestions tentatively since they would represent an extension of existing practice, rather than the reproduction of existing practice in other settings.

7 *The offering of alternative sources of satisfaction to junior staff*

Several commentators have detected a tendency for therapeutic communities to exploit junior staff (Manning, 1976b; Haddon, 1979). Therapeutic communities are 'greedy institutions' (Coser, 1974) which depend on a continual through-put of young, short-stay, idealistic staff who provide much of the day-to-day contact with residents. Consider this job description of the female 'social therapists' (in effect, short-term nursing assistants) employed in Maxwell Jones's pioneering hospital community:

> In selecting them, the Unit staff stress the importance of their being relatively healthy emotionally, attractive, intelligent, of responsive temperament and interested in people. These requirements are surprisingly like those of airline hostesses.... Scandinavians are thought to be especially suitable for the job of social therapist, not only for their physical attractiveness, but because of their 'democratic' approach. They do not typically relate to patients in terms of formal status differences as is so common among many British nurses. Their lack of nursing training is thought to facilitate this egalitarian approach. Being foreigners, formally untrained and transient, they are thought to have a lot in common with the patient. (Rapoport, 1967, p. 109)

In some communities particular features of the treatment approach might put a brake on this propensity towards exploiting junior staff. At Ashley the burdens of the staff role were perhaps eased by the stipulation that all staff should only take that degree of responsibility for the smooth running of the house that might reasonably be expected of an ordinary community member (the 'minimal supervisory role' described in Chapter 3). Further, a premium was placed on 'honest' relations with residents, and staff were not expected to dissemble their exasperation and annoyance.

The founding co-workers at Parkneuk had all worked previously in Camphill communities (where there is a large through-put of short-term co-workers) and out of those experiences had been born a determination to find ways of sustaining co-workers in post on a long-term basis. It was insisted that all co-workers should have the opportunity to develop alternative interests and find additional satisfaction in alternative pursuits within the organisational framework of the community. If a co-worker developed an interest in bee-keeping, then the community would agree to buy the hives and necessary equipment at a local 'roup' (farm auction sale). If a co-worker became interested in trying to dry the herbs grown in the community's field, then the community would agree to building a drying shed for the experiment. If a co-worker became interested in Khaki Campbells (egg-laying ducks), then these too could be obtained.

This incorporation of co-worker's leisure interests into the community 'programme' also provided an alternative career pathway for co-workers. Thus one couple left with a boarder to found a bio-dynamic herb and flower growing and drying business. As we pointed out in Chapter 1, a number of ex-Camphill co-workers who no longer wished to live and work in communal settings have set up houses and 'alternative' businesses whose uncertain earning power is boosted by the fees for taking in boarders on a short-term (school holidays) or long-term basis. If the kind of facilities at Parkneuk for training co-workers in crafts were extended to other communities, then the present trickle of junior staff into family fostering could become a steady flow. Under these circumstances an extensive family fostering system for psychiatric patients and the mentally handicapped might be feasible. In depopulated rural areas sufficient fosterers might be attracted by the availability of housing, workshops and land to allow a Geel-type development with similar clinical and nursing back-up facilities.

Self-evidently, communities such as Parkneuk are well-placed to develop staff craft skills, being residential for both staff and residents, and having task-oriented programmes. Nevertheless, many communities organise 'work groups' which could be planned to cater for staff as well as residents' needs. And even communities such as halfway houses, where many residents are absent during the day, are much exercised by the need to channel residents' energies into creative leisure pursuits.

We suspect that our overall approach to therapeutic practice, seeing it as a process of reality construction, will have an air of familiarity to many practitioners: our phenomenological approach has affinities with that found in the work of one of the greatest modern psychotherapists, Carl Rogers (1951). Practitioners may therefore derive greater interest from our descriptions of contrasting practices than from our theoretical framework. In this concluding section we have tried to sharpen this interest by drawing attention to particular practices which *may* be capable of further application in an increased number of settings.

Sociological implications

Although sociologists have frequently been allowed access to treatment settings, they have normally chosen to examine practitioners' conduct rather than practitioners' work. They have watched therapists (doctors, nurses, and other professionals) in the throes of the temporal construction of clinical cases, the complex processes of history-taking, examination, and intervention. But they have watched with tunnel vision. They retired to their offices to write reports, not on cognition, decision-making, or task-performance, but on, say, doctor-patient communication, patient satisfaction, or the control of patients. (We know what we're talking about – we have ourselves contributed to some of this literature: for example, Bloor, 1976). Such reports did not address what practitioners themselves saw as the core features of their everyday activities.

There were some early exceptions to this sociological neglect of the topic of medical work (for example, Fletcher, 1974), but, generally speaking, sociologists have been less interested in this topic than their colleagues in allied disciplines. In the philosophy of science there has long been a concern with the conceptualisation of clinical interpretation and intervention (see King, 1954, for an early example). More recently, interpretative anthropologists have broadened their interest from ethnographic studies of non-western healers to kindred studies of western medicine (Kleinman, 1980; Good and Good, 1980; Good et al., 1985). Physicians use clinical paradigms to guide their investigation of a patient's condition, beginning with complaints and symptoms, and interpreting them as the result of an underlying pathology, but Good and Good see this interpretative process as essentially similar to that universally used to understand particular phenomena in the light of scientific or popular models and to construct illness realities. Most influential of all have been the historical studies of Foucault, particularly his study of the growth of the French 'cliniques' at the end of the eighteenth century, where the French clinicians evolved a new language of seeing – the 'clinical gaze' – which reflexively both described and constructed the body as an invariable biological reality, and which remains the foundation of modern medical knowledge (Foucault, 1973; Armstrong, 1983, ix).

Influenced no doubt by all this extra-disciplinary activity, medical sociologists are now showing a similar interest in medical work. A notable recent example is Strauss et al.'s study (encompassing almost as many treatment settings as ours) of the organisation of medical work in different Californian hospitals (Strauss et al., 1985). It is in the context of this newly developed sociological interest in medical work that we wish to place the present study.

We have treated medical work in therapeutic communities as redefinitional work, the transformation of mundane events in the light of some paradigm of therapy. Like the anthropologists mentioned earlier, we would see a common thread of redefinitional activity running through all medical work, whether it be carried out by professionals or laymen, in surgeries, in hospitals, or in therapeutic communities. Redefinitions, or interpretations, may differ in their content but the redefinitional process itself possesses certain common properties.

To place our study in the context of a sociological perspective on medical work requires us to shift our emphasis from the description of diversity in therapeutic work to the identification of what hitherto has been only implicit in our analysis, namely, what we take to be the common properties of therapeutic work. These common properties do not have fixed values: they are not some lowest common denominator of diverse practices, or a residuum of similarity surrounded by a mass of diversity. Rather they are (with one exception) common dimensions of variability, universally present while differentially extensible. The different extensibility of these common properties allows us to map different approaches to therapeutic work in different settings. Accordingly, they may be useful for other students of medical work who may wish to make comparisons across different settings.

We shall consider in turn six formal properties or principles of therapeutic work. These principles are that therapeutic work is reflexive, interpretative, dominating, selective, and subject to habituation. We shall show how each of these principles except the first is differentially extensible, so that the different communities in our study may be distinguished in terms of such variance. Finally, we will consider the merits of our conceptualisation of therapeutic work relative to other conceptualisations found in the sociological literature.

1 Reflexivity

Reflexivity is not a differentially extensible property of therapeutic work: it is universal and invariate. By reflexivity we refer to the process whereby an utterance constitutes the reality it purports to describe, whereby an act of cognition constitutes the reality it seeks to apprehend. The reflexive character of all medical activity is well illustrated by King's elegant rhetorical question on medical discoveries:

> Does a disease, whatever it is, have a real existence, somehow, in its own right, in the same way as the continent of Australia? Such real existence would be independent of its discovery by explorer or investigator. A disease exists whether we know it or not. The contrasting point of view would hold that a disease is created by the inquiring intellect, carved out by the process of classification, in the same way that a statue is carved out of a block of marble by the chisel strokes of the sculptor. (King, 1954, p. 201).

In a similar way therapists' redefinitions are carved out of Schutz's undifferentiated horizon of thematic possibilities. The ethnomethodological convention of referring to activities as 'accomplishments' is an apt way of signalling the necessarily creative character of even the most repetitious acts. We do not seek to argue an extreme idealist position here: from a Schutzian standpoint any redefinition that is adopted and endorsed (rather than being discussed or aborted in the course of formulation) will be possessed of and shaped by considerations of pragmatic utility. Accomplished redefinitions may be various and even contradictory but they are not arbitrary or capricious.

We choose to stress the reflexive character of redefinitional work because of our previous emphasis on the reality-constructing nature of therapy. The treatment process is a process of reality construction: residents learn new and less pathogenic forms of social behaviour. The necessary reflexivity of redefinitions is the engine of reality construction: mundane occurrences are not just described by a redefinition, they are also constructed (or re-constructed). Catch-phrases, like 'You can only keep it if you give it away' (concept house), or 'How do you feel about that?' (day hospital), assume greater analytical significance when it is realised that every such invitation to a resident to describe is also an invitation to construct. In every community (reality-confronting or instrumental) residents absorb osmotically a new language of thought and seeing, a language that finds within prosaic and unconsidered activities various new features and qualities, a language that (like any other language) does not just apprehend and describe but also constitutes in the very acts of apprehension and description.

2 *Interpretation*

Just as the 'clinical gaze' conceives of the symptom as the surface signifier of the underlying disease pattern, so also there is a 'therapeutic gaze' which *interprets* apprehended resident behaviour as the signifier or indicator of an underlying social or psychiatric problem.

The interpretation is not novel but is instead one of a class with which the member (staff or resident) was previously familiar. However, the member may be motivated to elaborate his or her interpretation and establish its individual deviations from type. In other words, interpretation in therapeutic work varies in the elaborateness of its treatment of a given topic: the more elaborate the typification then the more specific or particular will be the features of that typification (note we use the term 'elaborateness' to refer to the variable treatment of a single topic, and we use the term 'extensiveness' to refer to the variable treatment of multiple topics – the one term signifies depth of coverage, the other signifies breadth of coverage). Any given interpretation will only have that degree of elaborateness demanded by the member's purpose at hand. It may be that only a relatively unspecific interpretation is required in order for an appropriate response to be decided upon; where interpretations are communicated to other members the speaker can possibly appeal to the others to elaborate for themselves their own sense of the interpretation whilst the interpretation that is voiced is itself rather abbreviated. Recall that interpretations at Parkneuk in particular often had this abbreviated character, but within any one community (and for any one member in respect of any one topic) the elaborateness of interpretations would shift sharply with context. The review groups and staff groups established in some communities allowed the consensual collective elaboration of interpretations of behaviour which, were interpretation to take place solely in the fleeting context where the behaviour occurred, might otherwise have been only an ambiguous or inadequate guide to intervention. The member's purpose at hand establishes the degree of specificity required of the interpretation but in the situation of action the pursuit of an adequate interpretation may be cut short by, in Schutz's phrase, the intrusion of new topical relevances – the onset of more pressing therapeutic concerns, sudden changes in the member's purpose at hand.

Where a relatively elaborate interpretation is required then meaning is not grasped monothetically – in a flash – but polythetically: there is an enquiring gaze which processually and sequentially grasps and constructs the phenomenon under scrutiny. The process of enquiry is conducted with increasing certitude up to the point where meaning appears sufficiently clear to satisfy the member's purpose at hand. The interpretation is not therefore problematic: in most circumstances the interpretation appears a self-evident truth, albeit open in principle to modification or contradiction should new topically relevant material suggest a reappraisal.

3 *Intervention*

Interpretation may sometimes be idle, as it were, quite without any accompanying intervention – a viewpoint expressed but discarded in a staff review group, or a silent assessment interrupted by more pressing concerns. More frequently, however, it may be said that the therapeutic community practitioner gazes only to intervene. In communications between members the interpretation may be left implicit whilst members concentrate on settling the correct intervention – 'what he really needs is...'. Alternatively, interpretations may focus less on the behaviour of the subject than on the context in which their behaviour occurs: interpretations are devoted to mundane events as appropriate occasions for intervention.

The symbiotic linkage of interpretation and intervention may also occur where interpretations are relatively elaborate. Enquiries may be polythetically elaborated not only up to the point where meaning appears obvious, but to where the appropriate action also appears obvious to the member. The interpretation suggests the intervention because the member is familiar with the situation; once he or she has settled on an interpretation the member does not normally need to embark on another polythetic enquiry to establish the appropriate intervention.

Paired interpretations and interventions may be sequentially linked in series over the course of a resident's career. An interpretation suggests an intervention whose impact may be such as to suggest a further interpretation which in turn suggests a further intervention and so on.

Most importantly, in the light of all our previous discussion, intervention in therapeutic work can be divided into two types, partly complementary, partly competitive: on the one hand we have reality confrontation, reflecting views of the subject's behaviour back to the subject and making the subject the observer of his or her own activities; on the other hand, we have instrumentalism, dictating behavioural change by the engineering of the subject's social environment.

4 Domination

We take a Foucauldian view of power as a strategic relationship, a routine fact of life in therapeutic communities as elsewhere. Power is manifested in the near-continuous monitoring or surveillance that is a necessary pre-cursor of all redefinitions. The observing gaze of the therapist, like that of the clinician, creates a power relationship between the observer and the observed: 'the eye that knows and decides, the eye that governs' (Foucault, 1973, p. 89). Power cannot be abolished or legislated away, but dominance – manifested and felt imbalances and inequalities in that strategic relationship – varies.

Manifest power provokes resistance and, as we saw in Chapter 5, concealment was a frequent resident response to the therapeutic gaze. The degree of dominance will partly depend on how far such concealment and other techniques of resistance are successful. It will also partly depend on the techniques by which power is manifested.

Two manifestations of power which obviously contribute towards dominance are authority and social control. Authority is always a potential option in any power relationship, to be assumed if the superordinate so chooses. The option is more likely to be exercised in instrumental communities, but we have seen that some staff in reality-confronting communities might also take up an authoritative stance in order to provoke resident dissent (witness Dave's bellowing at Victor at Ashley). Likewise, social control or 'manipulation' (as some writers on power would have it – Lukes, 1974; Bachrach and Baratz, 1962) are also potential options to be exercised if a superordinate chooses. Elsewhere, Bloor (1986c) has disputed Sharp's argument that social control is an inevitable corollary of therapeutic work (Sharp, 1975). Bloor cites instances of therapeutic work being undertaken to provoke dissent as well as to overcome it, and of the deliberate tolerance of disruption as well as action to ensure the smooth running of the community; Bloor presents social control as simply one option for superordinates who may well choose instead to 'orchestrate' therapy – the planning and anticipation of events by superordinates without recourse to control by virtue of their skills and experience as therapists. Orchestration might almost be defined as the exercise of power without domination.

The nature of the therapeutic gaze itself may be a determinant of dominance. Foucault, writing of Bentham's prison design (the Panopticon), implied that domination was increased to the extent that surveillance was anonymous and disembodied. The pooling of information to form a collective staff view of residents, and the recording of the results of surveillance in residents' files, for example, could be seen as promoting an anonymous and disembodied staff gaze.

Where the therapist has an intensive living and working relationship with residents, then the gaze may seem far from disembodied. But the dissembling of surveillance under the cover of mundane activities (remember the staff member's periodic trips from the office to the laundry?) may serve, paradoxically, to increase residents' feelings of being subject to constant scrutiny once that cover is removed.

It follows that domination will vary from community to community as surveillance practices vary, and techniques of resident resistance and staff counteraction also vary. Some staff practices will tend to increase dominance (for example, the concept house practice of requiring fellow-residents to monitor and denounce residents' misdemeanours), whilst others will diminish it (for example, the Ashley practice of allowing residents access to their own reports).

5 *Selectivity*

Although any and every event and utterance in the therapeutic community is potentially open to redefinition, some selectivity must be exercised in the choice of topics as a consequence of the complexity and onrush of social life in the therapeutic community. The redefinition of one resident's difficulties must often be omitted, cut short, or postponed, to deal with the pressing requirements of another resident. The redefinition of tangential events must be sacrificed to the clarity of a main redefinitional theme. Allowance must be made for fatigue – fatigue of both the redefiner and the recipient. Expressed redefinitions may create situations requiring further redefinition which in turn may lead to further situations requiring redefinition, and so on – consuming time and resources without necessarily culminating in natural closure. And finally, if redefinitions are expressed, they may disrupt the routine activities on which they intrude. As we have seen, in some communities therapists attempt to create a naturalistic (rather than natural), family-like (rather than familial) regime of 'benign routines'. This regime requires periodic maintenance from staff; staff must monitor, interpret, and act upon events to promote and restore benign routines, but some selectivity must also be exercised in redefinitional work in order to protect routines. There is also the possibility that the enmeshment of members in benign routines such as meal preparation may lead to a partial loss of reflectivity (see below) or to the ritualistic elevation of task-completion over the practice of therapy.

Just as we have previously seen that the extensibility of interpretations will vary both within and between communities, so also the same variation applies to the *topics* of interpretation – selectivity occurs both within and between communities.

6 Habituation

Particular interpretations may become what Schutz has termed 'habitual possessions' (Schutz, 1970), assimilated into the therapist's stock of knowledge at hand (perhaps at a given level of extensiveness and specificity) and readily available for matching and articulation under appropriate typified circumstances.

Habituation results in a telescoping of the polythetic search process described earlier, so that we could treat habituation as mere loss of interpretation were it not for the fact that we also see habituation in intervention and in selectivity. However, any such curtailing of the search-process is unlikely to result in a shift from the polythetic to the monothetic mode of cognition, where meaning is grasped subliminally and reaction takes place unthinkingly and as a matter of course; it may well be a relevant pursuit for the therapist to inspect phenomena in respect of their deviation(s) from his habitual possessions.

We could add more properties of therapeutic work, and indeed, additional properties might be abstracted from the foregoing discussion, for example, the sequential – or temporally ordered – character of therapeutic work, the naturalistic location of therapeutic work, and so on. But they would lack the salience of our existing list.

One of the properties on our list (reflexivity) refers to the reality-constructing character of the treatment process. The remaining five properties represent, not invariate qualities, but dimensions of variability: areas of difference within which various types of therapeutic community can be located and mapped – witness the reality-confronting interventions of Ashley versus the instrumentalism of Beeches, the benign routine (habituation) of Parkneuk versus the 'pressure cooker' of the concept house, the relative domination exercised at the concept house and at Ashley, and so on.

Other conceptual approaches

Ours is not the first sociological study of medical work in general or therapeutic work in particular. Some alternative approaches have been touched on earlier; we can note five in all:

Strauss et al.'s 'illness trajectories'

Foucault's 'clinical gaze'

therapeutic work as synonymous with members' accounts of their activities (Rawlings, 1980, 1981)

a mechanism for the social control of residents (Sharp, 1975)

an institutional rhetoric serving to influence the relationships between the community and powerful outside agencies (Walter, 1978).

We have not the space here to discuss all these approaches as fully as they deserve and we have already commented upon some of them at length elsewhere (Bloor, 1986c; Bloor and McKeganey, 1986). Accordingly, we provide only summary comment on the last three authors and confine our detailed discussion to the first two approaches.

Respecting the work of Sharp and Walter, we fully accept that therapeutic work can be used as a mechanism of social control (Sharp) and as a device for impression management in dealings with outside agencies (Walter). We accept that therapeutic work *can* have such uses, but we dispute that it is confined to such uses. For example, we have ourselves observed the use of redefinitions to maintain social control of residents, but we have also observed the deliberate tolerance of disruption and the planned provocation of resident dissent, both for avowed therapeutic purposes.

Respecting the ethnomethodological approach, it will be clear that our own work has been much influenced by ethnomethodological studies (witness our discussion of reflexivity), and Fonkert's original research was in fact conceived as an ethnomethodological study. However, our topic in this book is a 'substantive' one, the comparative description of therapeutic work. As ethnomethodologists have repeatedly pointed out to puzzled critics, ethnomethodological studies do not have substantive topical foci – their concern is with members' methods, with the methods that collectivity members use to constitute and order their social reality as a taken-for-granted facticity (Mehan and Wood, 1975). This is not to say that such studies cannot make important incidental contributions to substantive topics (see Hester, 1981), but by definition no ethnomethodological study would *focus* on a topic such as ours. Conceptual differentiation may arise out of differentiation of topic: we would not expect a study of members' methods to share our concern with the differential extensibility of properties of therapeutic work across different communities.

Although the research of Strauss and his colleagues on medical work was first reported in 1979 (Wiener et al., 1979), we confess it was not until their book had been published in 1985 and our own work was nearing completion that we realised the degree of similarity between their approach and our own. They too perceived a lacuna in the sociological conception of work:

> . . .remarkably little writing in the sociology of work begins with work itself (except descriptively, not analytically) but rather focuses on the divisions of labour, on work roles, role relationships, careers, and the like. (Strauss et al., p. xi)

In response to this lacuna they focused on what they termed 'illness trajectories':

> . . .trajectory is a term coined . . . to refer not only to the physiological unfolding of a patient's disease but to the total organisation of work done over that course, plus the impact on those involved with that work and its organisation. For different illnesses, the trajectory will involve different medical and nursing actions, different kinds of skills and other resources, a different parcelling out of tasks among the workers (including, perhaps, kin and the patient), and involving quite different relationships – instrumental and expressive both – among the workers. (Strauss et al., p. 8)

An illness trajectory thus provides an organising framework for the depiction of medical work which stresses the sequential ordering and interdependence of tasks. Strauss et al. proceed to discuss particular types of tasks such as 'machine work', 'comfort work', and so on.

The main difference between our two approaches seems to us to lie with the emphasis Strauss and his colleagues place on work as task performance compared to our emphasis on work as an act of cognition. Indeed it may seem, to some practitioners, rather perverse of us to describe therapeutic work as an act of cognition, especially when the practitioner has been largely involved all day in manhandling caravans or digging pea trenches. Strauss and his colleagues, in contrast, simply treat cognitive acts as further species of tasks, in particular the first and second levels of 'articulation work' (Strauss et al., pp. 155–156).

However, this difference between the two approaches seems to us readily explicable and reasonable in view of the contrasting objectives of the two studies. Strauss et al. have conceived of medical work as having an essential structure and procedure that is native to any work or enterprise: 'any enterprise ... can usefully be conceived of as a trajectory, with its arc of work and implicated tasks.' (Strauss et al., p. 290). They have produced a sociological description of hospital work as an exemplar of the sociology of work. In contrast, we have sought to emphasise how any enterprise can be singled out and accounted as therapeutic work: we are concerned with the transformative redefinition of tasks into therapy. Strauss and his colleagues are concerned with the sociology of work and have elegantly demonstrated how general features of work may be found in particular tasks. We are concerned with the sociology of therapeutic work in therapeutic communities and have focused on the cognitive acts whereby practitioners distinguish therapeutic work amidst undifferentiated mundane tasks.

In setting ourselves this more limited objective our study is more akin to Foucault's analysis of the 'clinical gaze', where Foucault set himself the task of describing what was distinctive about the new approach to medical practice found in the French cliniques. Other authors have found much in Foucault's work which can be reapplied to areas of contemporary medical practice (see especially Armstrong, 1983). Despite our pious protestations of limited objectives, we would naturally be best pleased to have our cake and eat it. We have not developed our conceptualisation of therapeutic work as an exemplar (as have Strauss and his colleagues), but we believe that there may be parallels that can be drawn between therapeutic work in therapeutic communities and other areas of the medical enterprise. However, we must leave the establishment of such parallels to future empirical investigation by other researchers.

Our work has been influenced in part by Foucault, so our assertion of similarities between the 'clinical gaze' and 'therapeutic work' will hardly be surprising. In the main, these similarities are fortuitous rather than engineered: it was our realisation that therapeutic work consisted in the transformative redefinition of mundane activities that led us to formulate therapeutic work as cognitive activity rather than, say, a speech act or task performance. Similarly, although Foucault refers to the 'gaze' or the 'surveillance' of the clinician he does not imply a purely physical, ocular activity: the clinical gaze is first and foremost a cognitive activity. As a consequence, several of our properties of therapeutic work are also writ large in Foucault's formulation: the clinical gaze is also interpretative and reflexive – the clinician apprehends symptoms as the surface signifier of the disease pattern, constructing the illness in the act of apprehension.

The similarity of the clinical gaze and therapeutic work is an engineered similarity in respect of the property of domination. It was only through Foucault's work (particularly Foucault, 1980) that we came to appreciate with any clarity the exercise of power in therapeutic work, and that domination is engendered by surveillance. Our ascription of domination as a property of therapeutic work is testimony to Foucault's influence.

We are uncertain whether Foucault's gaze can be considered interventionist in the sense found in therapeutic work. This may reflect some ambiguity in Foucault's work. On the one hand, Foucault stresses that the gaze is prior to, and distinct from, intervention: 'the observing gaze refrains from intervening: it is silent and gestureless' (Foucault, 1973, p. 107); and again, 'this gaze ... which refrains from all possible intervention' (*ibid.*, p. 108). On the other hand, as Armstrong has pointed out (in a personal communication), the dialectical relationship of interpretation and intervention in therapeutic work is also found in Foucault's writings: the surgeon and the pathologist both intervene in order to observe.

We are on more certain ground when we consider the differential extensibility of our properties of therapeutic work, as this was not an aspect of the clinical gaze which it was Foucault's purpose to consider. Foucault was not concerned to map differences in practice between different French cliniques. He was concerned rather to contrast the practices of these cliniques *as a group* with what had gone before; his clinical gaze is an idealisation unconcerned with imperfections in realisation or failures in execution.

Accordingly, the clinical gaze is conceived of as an exhaustive scan of accessible reality: selectivity of observation is not practised. Nor are the glossing, abbreviation, and appeals to the obvious (which we relate to habituation) found in Foucault's analysis. Differential selectivity and habituation are properties responsive to the practical exigencies of therapeutic community practice and these practical exigencies were not Foucault's concern – indeed one would not expect them to be well reported in the historical sources that formed Foucault's data.

The same arguments apply to the differential extensibility of interpretations, intervention, and domination: comparisons between cliniques were not part of Foucault's design and so the clinical gaze could be ascribed invariate properties rather than properties representing dimensions of difference. Moreover, it is possible that Foucault's sources inadequately represented such variations in extensibility as occurred, just as today's textbooks on diagnosis represent idealisations of practice rather than being grounded in empirical descriptions of contextualised diagnostic procedures.

In short, our conceptualisation of therapeutic work has much in common with Foucault's 'clinical gaze'. That it has not more in common is largely due to the fact that Foucault's concept is not designed to map variations in practice. To the extent that our concept is so designed, it may be of some use to other researchers.

As we emphasised at the beginning of this chapter, we have no wish to stipulate the sociological implications that others may draw from our analysis. Some may see most value in our depiction of how differential access among staff to information about patients may influence therapeutic effectiveness (see Chapter 6). Others may be more interested in our attempts to describe local techniques of power and resistance (see Chapter 5). But we would certainly hope that the conceptual approach adopted here will be of some use to other sociologists who may wish to compare and contrast medical work across different organisational settings.

For the general reader

The main interest of therapeutic communities for a general readership probably lies in their appearance as a social movement, and in their influence on social change – actual and potential. As sociologists we have no licence to make authoritative pronouncements on such a topic, and it is right for us to make clear here that our rather Wellsian statements at the end of Chapter 1 (on the contemporary outlook for therapeutic communities) were no more than the speculations of informed outsiders. Authoritative pronouncements on social change are the business of social critics, not sociologists.

One social critic has stood pre-eminent in recent years in his denunciation of the medical enterprise in general and the therapeutic relationship in particular. We refer to Ivan Illich. When Illich turned his attention to the iatrogenic effects of medicine he brought with him a considerable reputation from his previous libertarian criticisms of development aid and compulsory schooling. There were considerable sales for *Medical Nemesis* (Illich, 1975) and its revised successor *Limits to Medicine* (Illich, 1977), and lengthy, respectful reviews in publications like the *British Medical Journal.* Illich believes professional health care systems to be creating sickness in three ways – by clinical iatrogenesis, the creation of sickness and death by medical intervention; by social iatrogenesis, the generation of an addictive demand for medical goods and services; and by structural iatrogenesis, the expropriation of the power of individuals and collectivities to heal themselves (Illich, 1975, p. 165).

Illich argues that the only answer to iatrogenesis is demedicalisation, a political consensus in favour of the curtailment of the output of medical goods and services and the reassertion of family and neighbourhood responsibility for health and sickness. This is not a popular argument, even among those who share Illich's concern about iatrogenesis. To many, Illich's demedicalisation seems uncomfortably close to government 'community care' policies which herd ex-psychiatric hospital patients into redundant seaside boarding houses and which trap wives and mothers into traditional 'unpaid carer' roles. In this last section we look at how far therapeutic communities may represent institutional alternatives to demedicalisation – non-iatrogenic approaches to health-care, institutional locales for the reassertion of individual and collective responsibility for care and cure.

At hardly any point in our analysis so far have we found all therapeutic communities occupying the same ground in respect of a given proposition. A similar pattern of variation emerges when we consider therapeutic communities and the reduction of structural iatrogenesis.

It is clear that Illich would approve of communities such as Geel, which substitute natural relations of family and neighbourhood care for psychiatric hospital treatment, and where boarders can derive satisfaction from relations of mutual aid and from their contribution to the domestic economy of the host family. Parkneuk and our Camphill community might share this approbation insofar as their practices of promoting 'benign routines' (Parkneuk) and 'permissive instrumentalism' (Camphill) show some affinities with the Geel foster family approach (see Chapter 2). We see no reason to suppose that the healing power of family relations is expropriated when these relations are transferred from Belgian household to Scottish institution.

The position of the reality-confronting communities (Faswells, Ravenscroft, Ashley, and the day hospital) requires fuller consideration. we can note three aspects of the treatment approach in such communities which might serve to reduce iatrogenesis – the conception of residents' problems as lying in social relationships and behaviour, the emphasis on collective responsibility for treatment, and the volitional character of behavioural change. To establish how these aspects of the treatment approach may reduce iatrogenesis we need to be clearer on how structural iatrogenesis is produced.

In the course of an extraordinarily vituperative review of Illich's *Medical Nemesis* (Illich is aligned, at different points, with Milton Friedman, ex-President Nixon and the Woodstock hippies) Vicente Navarro, the Marxist clinician, equates structural iatrogenesis with alienation. The equation is probably a correct one (Illich himself does not use the term 'alienation'), provided we restrict our sense of the term to that found in the young, Hegelian Marx. The young Marx gives the word various shades of meaning in different contexts, but a satisfactory summary definition encompasses three necessary components: first, a process of externalisation or objectification; second, a loss of control of the externalised object; and third, the experiencing of the externalised object as an instrument of oppression:

> His labour becomes an object, assumes an external existence. . . . it exists independently outside himself, i.e. outside his control and alien to him, and . . . stands opposed to him as autonomous power. (Marx, 1963, pp. 122–3).

There is an arresting parallel between the processes leading to the alienation of the worker and those leading to the alienation of the patient: in the course of medical treatment the patients' illnesses and disabilities become 'thingified' objects, and in this separation patients experience a loss of control and find their illness standing over and above them, an instrument of constraint and oppression. Such alienation seems inherent in the very processes of doctor-patient relations in professional and bureaucratised medical care systems, rather than being a feature of the control and use of these systems (Bloor and Harris, 1984).

Thus the processes of medical diagnosis and treatment in most clinical settings reconstruct the patient's complaint as a biological abstraction, disregarding the patient's environment and social and productive activity (Wartofsky, 1974). Such disregard, as Strong (1979) points out, may be in the cause of that moral neutrality that accompanies bureaucratically regulated activity, but this same disregard for the patient's sociality constructs the illness as a remote and separate object. In the therapeutic community a more holistic approach operates; the community is a *speculum mundi* wherein the resident's problems may be located as part and parcel of that resident's everyday social behaviour – the 'problem' is no abstracted biological malfunction, but integral to the resident's social world.

Just as labour becomes an alien activity to the worker – he is not at home in his work and avoids it when possible – so also the patient role is an alien activity to the patient undergoing conventional medical treatment. There is no self-realisation in being the passive recipient of professional and bureaucratised medical care. In most treatment settings the patient is obligated only to wish to get well and follow the prescribed medical regimen (Parsons, 1964, pp. 274–5). In therapeutic communities residents are obligated to take an active part in their own treatment. This is a collective as well as an individual patient responsibility. In conventional medical care settings the individual patient has no responsibilities for the care of others. Like Marx's alienated worker he becomes monadic and egotistic, withdrawn into his own suffering. In the therapeutic community lay care is given new significance and worth.

Finally, just as control of the product of the worker's labour passes to the capitalist, so control of the objectified illness passes to medical professionals in conventional treatment settings. The patient's condition becomes an instrument of the patient's domination, and there are many studies which show long-term patients contesting this loss of control and adopting various strategies to influence their regimens (Roth, 1963, Braginsky et al., 1969). In reality-confronting communities behaviour change is an act of volition exercised by the resident.

So in three aspects – a holistic conception of residents' problems, individual and collective responsibility for treatment, and the volitional character of treatment – reality-confronting communities can be seen to reduce iatrogenesis. Yet this must be set against the evidence cited in Chapter 5 of a power contest in therapeutic communities, of staff surveillance and resident resistance. Under these circumstances reality-confronting communities may not be wholly free of a tendency towards producing structural iatrogenesis. But, as we have seen, there are different degrees of domination and these communities may be judged considerably less iatrogenic than alternative treatments.

We have left till last Beeches and the concept house. Both these communities attempted resocialisation not by volition (as in the reality-confronting communities) but by unremarked assimilation and by sanctioning. To be sure, a holistic view of residents' problems is retained, and residents are not isolated but drawn into the resocialisation of fellow residents. However, those readers who endorse Illich's libertarian perspective may feel that the programming of residents for behavioural change is self-evidently an expropriation (Illich's term) of residents' power to heal themselves, since it removes the pivot around which such power could be exercised: it removes the element of choice.

Many therapeutic communities (but not all) thus represent institutional alternatives to those conventional patterns of medical consumption identified and denounced by Illich. Therapeutic communities offer therapeutic relationships without a passive dependency on professional staff: residents actively collaborate in their own treatment. Further, the dyadic professional-client relationship disappears as the resident culture becomes an agency of therapy and residents participate in one another's treatment. Viewed in this way, therapeutic communities might well be thought to stand with one foot in Eden.

Appendix
Research methods

Introduction

This appendix is really two methods appendices rolled into one. The first part is meant to be used for reference purposes by those readers interested in particular aspects of our methodology – the choice of study topic, the choice of study settings, the methods of data collection and the methods of data analysis. We shall try to keep this part as brief as possible in order to allow ourselves space for the second part of the appendix, in which we concentrate on our experiences as participant observers in therapeutic communities. Here we discuss the ways in which our awareness and understanding of events was seemingly influenced by our social status in the communities we studied – not just by our marginal role and temporary engagement, but by our social relationships with community members and by those statuses ascribed by gender and age of which the researcher may, at times, be only partially aware (du Boulay and Williams, 1987). We also reflect here on the ways in which events and experiences in our study communities influenced us in turn and impinged not just on our effectiveness as researchers, but also on our personal lives outside the setting and after the fieldwork was completed.

Choice of topic and settings

We have already recounted how our various research settings were themselves the focus of individual studies. Fieldwork had already been conducted in three settings and was beginning in a fourth when we made a definite commitment to undertake a comparative study of the range of therapeutic community practice. At that time, Bloor had completed one study (of Parkneuk) and was writing up a second (of the day hospital) as part of a wider programme of research on de-institutionalisation at the Medical Research Council's Medical Sociology Unit. McKeganey was conducting postgraduate research at the MRC unit on an ESRC studentship linked to Bloor's work; he was just starting fieldwork at a Camphill community. Fonkert had completed his thesis on the concept house and, having married a British nurse, had moved to Britain to look for academic employment. Fonkert and Bloor had become aware of each other's work through a mutual academic acquaintance (Harley Frank) and discovered a good deal of common ground: they had both employed participant observation methods and both envisaged the treatment process as a process of reality construction.

All three of us met to discuss the possibility of pooling our respective resources for a retrospecive comparative analysis in 1980. While we agreed that the project was worthwhile, we all felt that the comparative study would have a greater appeal if we could make some claim to have encompassed the range of therapeutic community practice. Inevitably this meant 'theoretical sampling' of certain additional contrasting types of therapeutic community, at a minimum a halfway house and a residential psychiatric treatment unit. It was clear that the way to proceed in these further settings was on the basis of our previous work, that is, to focus each of the additional studies on discrete topics which could attract funding in their own right, but to frame them in such a way that they could fit neatly into our comparative study. At this time we also 'piloted' the feasibility of a retrospective comparison by comparing the process of reality construction in two of our communities – the day hospital and the concept house (Bloor and Fonkert, 1982).

Bloor approached a charitable trust well known for its network of halfway house therapeutic communities and, on discovering that its various houses covered a wide range of practice, suggested a comparison of two similarly circumstanced houses ('Ashley' and 'Beeches') which employed contrasting approaches to therapy. Support for this work was provided by the Medical Research Council and the charitable trust agreed to waive the usual rent for the researcher's accommodation.

On completion of McKeganey's thesis, he and Bloor put together a grant application for a study of the impact on therapeutic work in residential communities of external constraints associated with their hospital location – a topic which, though much discussed in the practitioner literature, was largely unresearched. Initially, the study was framed as focusing on one representative community (Faswells) identified by officers of the Association of Therapeutic Communities. Funding was eventually secured from the Economic and Social Research Council, one of whose referees suggested including a second community (Ravenscroft) as a way of checking on the actual representativeness of Faswells. As it turned out, we were most grateful for this advice since, although the two communities were experiencing similar constraints, it was only at Faswells that these had supposedly led to any erosion of the treatment programme.

In focusing the broader comparative study on a description of everyday practice within and across our various communities, we managed to combine our sociological interests in medical work and reality construction with practitioners' natural curiosity about practices in other communities. Nevertheless, many of the practitioners we have been in contact with would probably have preferred us to have conducted a conventional evaluative assessment of their work. Reasons for this are not hard to find: in their dealings with referral agencies, funding agencies, and administrators, practitioners are acutely aware of the political clout associated with a scientifically reputable study demonstrating the effectiveness of their communities. However, there are insuperable problems associated with studying a service as if it were a drug, most of which have been expounded elsewhere (notably in Illsley, 1980). In the first place, as will have been obvious from even the most cursory examination of this book, therapeutic communities vary enormously in their approach to treatment, in their clientele, in their typical length of resident careers, and in their views of success and failure. No evaluation study of a single community could possibly produce results relevant to the evaluation of all communities. To produce generalisable findings a study would have to take a multi-centred approach, which with the addition of more than a few communities would become prohibitively expensive, and would still be open to the criticism that the sampled communities were different from the unsampled communities in ways which were possibly crucial to successful practice.

Second, it is simply not possible to produce universal criteria of success that could be unproblematically applied across communities. Readmission rates have been a popular criterion, but in some communities (such as the concept houses) departure and readmission may be stages in a continuing process of treatment. There are standardised psychiatric screening instruments which may minimise observer variation in assessments, but none of these can be employed, grid-like, across the range of problems (mental handicap at Camphill, addiction at the concept house, and so on) catered for by different communities.

Third, it is unlikely that any researcher would be able to ensure random allocation of residents between communities and alternative, competing treatment regimes. Also, admission policies vary across institutions and many communities screen out less motivated applicants (this is a problem with the concept house studies), or else exclude unsuitable residents at an early stage of treatment. For various reasons, then, the researcher may end up comparing resident performance between different treatment regimes, each of which have selected their resident populations on quite different grounds and do not therefore bear comparison.

Finally, control trial studies require large numbers of subjects for statistical analysis. Communities with small numbers of residents (like Parkneuk), or a lengthy treatment programme (like Camphill) cannot readily be evaluated in this manner.

Therapeutic communities are not alone in presenting almost intractable problems for the design of evaluative studies; many institutions in the social and health services are in the same boat – with unstandardised inputs, heterogeneous clientele, small throughputs, and subjective assessment criteria. To continue to conduct conventional evaluative studies under these circumstances and claim a general applicability of findings is to indulge in 'scientism'; providing a spurious scientific gloss for necessary political decisions on resource allocation. In effect, a descriptive study of a range of therapeutic communities is not an alternative to controlled evaluation, it is the *only* viable research strategy. We have encompassed a wider range of settings than any evaluative study could embrace and we have deliberately focused on variations in practice – depicting therapeutic community practice as varying along specific continua. To compare and contrast variations in practice is itself highly relevant to evaluation and, for some types of service provision, may be the closest one can come to evaluation.

Data collection and analysis

For each of the component studies, descriptions of the techniques of data collection and analysis have already been published. We shall provide only a summary here, concentrating on differences in technique between the component studies. Most attention will be devoted to the reanalysis for the comparative study.

All the component studies were participant observer studies. In six of the settings (Ashley, Beeches, Faswells, Ravenscroft, Parkneuk and Camphill) the researchers adopted roles broadly akin to that of a junior staff member. At the concept house, Fonkert participated in the house 'structure' like an ordinary resident (staff were not part of the structure), although he had access to staff meetings and was not residential. At the day hospital, Bloor spent the first half of his fieldwork with the patients and the second half with the staff. We are not concerned at this point with our 'staff bias' in data-collection; it will be evident that a study of therapeutic work (and particularly a study that conceives of therapeutic work as an act of cognition!) must use methods that give access to staff thinking. Rather, we are interested in the comparability of the different data collected in the different settings. If there is any uncertainty here it must be over Fonkert's data and whether his participation as a resident led to divergence from the other studies. But we can dismiss this possibility: recall that the concept house, uniquely among therapeutic communities, sought to transform residents into staff, and in fact Fonkert later went on to work for some months as a staff member at a nearby day centre for addicts.

In all the study settings data were collected largely in the form of fieldnotes. In some settings additional materials were collected – documents, audio recordings of conversations and groups, of interviews, and of panel discussions. In only one instance were audio recordings used as a substitute for fieldnotes: at Faswells, McKeganey was refused direct access to the small groups as it was felt that his temporary presence would have a dislocating effect on relationships within the group; instead, each of the groups undertook to record their proceedings in his absence. In all other contexts at Faswells McKeganey relied on fieldnotes.

Parenthetically, where direct access had been granted, we would not regard audio recordings as an acceptable substitute for fieldnotes in ethnography. Leaving aside the technical problems – such as those of recording, for example, in Parkneuk's (horticultural) field, or in their often noisy workshop – and leaving aside the considerable logistical problems of transcribing and analysing many hours of recordings, we agree with Hammersley and Atkinson (1983) that the ethnographer is his or her own research instrument. The tape recorder is a 'cultural dope' and is of only supplementary value for an ethnographer.

We had hoped to undertake a *systematic* reanalysis of our data for the comparative study; in the event we had to settle for a much more ad hoc arrangement. It had been envisaged that the authors would sketch out a set of agreed themes for the comparative study and then jointly develop an index of topics associated with these themes. All the data would be re-indexed (several of the component studies had already entailed individual indexing systems), possibly using a computerised indexing system, and analysis would proceed by an 'analytic induction' approach (Bloor, 1978) – the development of propositions for each separate indexed topic by comparative consideration of all the indexed fieldnotes relating to that topic. It didn't work out like that.

The last component studies were completed and written up in 1985. By that time Fonkert had returned to Holland and was working long hours in non-academic employment, McKeganey had embarked on the itinerant 'career' of the contract researcher and Bloor's research unit was being relocated to Glasgow with a new research programme – not a very promising scenario for a systematic reanalysis.

We had to adopt a much more limited and ad hoc approach. (This is not meant apologetically: we are rather proud of our achievement in completing any comparative analysis at all.) Bloor and McKeganey were both able (thanks to understanding directors) to analyse and write up material on a part-time basis whilst also working on other projects. Fonkert had provided an English translation of his dissertation but had little opportunity for more extensive participation. Bloor and McKeganey divided up between themselves primary responsibility for the various book chapters. Each took responsibility for two of the four chapters reporting empirical data; two of those chapters (3 and 6) involved the elaboration of themes already explored in component studies, but the remaining two chapters could not be based on previous analyses. Each chapter took shape rather differently and presented different analytical and literary problems; for example, the main problem we faced in Chapter 3 was the length of the first draft and how to reduce it by about half without the loss of thematically relevant material.

A natural history of the analysis and write-up of each chapter would presume an unlikely, and perhaps even unnatural, degree of reader interest. Yet the question of how studies, particularly those involving a number of researchers, are written up is an important one. We shall compromise here and provide a resumé of the production of one specimen chapter – Chapter 5.

Chapter 5 was the chapter least adequately conceived in early plans. Initially it was decided to focus the chapter on a number of topics bearing upon the selection of events for redefinitional work within and across our communities. We aimed to look at the audience to whom redefinitions were provided, the content of these redefinitions and the degree of their specificity. Perhaps partly because of this initial vagueness, Bloor and McKeganey also felt that this would be a logical place for a discussion of power and resident resistance.

Bloor argued for conceiving of power in Foucauldian terms since this would allow them to focus on 'local strategies' of power and resistance. McKeganey accepted the suggestion and agreed to take primary responsibility for the chapter. However, he felt that Bloor would be better placed to produce a first draft of the section on power. With this decided, McKeganey began working on the first part of the chapter, and Bloor reviewed his Ashley and Beeches data, in which resident resistance had been one of the indexed items. The inductive typology of strategies of resident resistance outlined in Chapter 5 was developed in relation to these two communities, with the day hospital and Parkneuk data being reviewed for comparable and contrasting material.

McKeganey, however, was unhappy with the work on his part of the chapter. As a result of pressure from other commitments, he had attempted to telescope the separate spheres of analysis and write-up, and in the process unwittingly created a situation in which he had begun writing without any clear idea of where the chapter was going – a disheartening experience. Bloor handed his fieldnotes over to McKeganey who, armed with these, but not Fonkert's (only the dissertation had been translated), pulled both parts of the chapter together and handed Bloor a completed first draft. Bloor's reaction mirrored McKeganey's own disappointment – to both of them it seemed the chapter was going over ground already covered elsewhere in the book. With the expiry of one publisher's deadline the space for manoeuvre was slight; the choice, it seemed, was between dropping the chapter entirely (something neither really wanted to see happen) or refocusing the chapter on that one section of the first draft which they had both liked: a discussion of variations in the selection of the audience for redefinitional work within and across the communities.

In the course of weighing these options Bloor recalled a paper on Barbadian 'dropped remarks' (Fisher, 1976) referred to at a conference he had attended some months previously. McKeganey agreed with Bloor that the dropped remark device was highly relevant within the therapeutic community context where audience selection was a salient concern. The chapter, then, would be recast in more of a sociolinguistic vein, addressing the issue of audience selection. It was obvious that this refocusing would not sit particularly comfortably with the section on power, but the authors were long past the point of caring about such niceties.

McKeganey set to reviewing his and Bloor's data with this issue in mind. By pulling out those instances where redefinitions were provided, McKeganey could look at the question of audience. Fairly quickly it was apparent that the data could be divided between those occasions when residents were the typical audience (such as at Faswells and Ravenscroft) and those where staff were the typical audience (such as at Camphill). It was apparent that the topic of audience selection bore closely upon our earlier distinction between those communities adopting a reality-confronting approach to therapy, and those where the approach was more instrumental. McKeganey decided to focus the chapter on the Faswells/Camphill contrast and began searching his data for deviant cases – situations in Faswells and Ravenscroft when staff were the audience for redefinitional accounts and situations in Camphill when the children were the audience.

Bloor had arranged to visit Fonkert in Holland for a long weekend to go over his reactions to the draft chapters. There was no point in showing Fonkert the already scrapped first draft of Chapter 5. Instead McKeganey prepared a list of questions for Bloor to ask Fonkert on the topics of audience and resident resistance in the concept house; Bloor also outlined to Fonkert their thinking on the two main themes of the chapter. Armed with Fonkert's (reported) answers, and having read through all of Bloor's fieldnotes for comparable and contrasting information on the topic of audience selection, McKeganey began the redrafting process. As far as the section on power was concerned, McKeganey accepted Bloor's typology of forms of resident resistance, but qualified and illustrated these in relation to his own communities. Finally, he pulled the two parts of the chapter together and handed Bloor a completed second draft. McKeganey and Bloor then went through Bloor's reactions to the second draft. It had seemed to Bloor that the chapter would profit from being more firmly located within the wider context of sociolinguistic discussions of audience selection and to this end he set out his thoughts on an alternative introduction. Bloor's remaining comments had to do with his feeling that the concentration on Faswells and Camphill had led McKeganey to under-emphasise what he, Bloor, took to be an important feature of staff work at Beeches, namely the exchange of redefinitions amongst staff in the service of producing a consensual case picture of residents, and of planning programmes of intervention. Both of these activities, though prominent at Beeches, were much less salient at Faswells and Camphill. McKeganey accepted Bloor's suggestions and made the necessary amendments to the chapter. With a mixture of relief and anxious anticipation the chapter was sent to Fonkert, who duly approved it.

This warts-and-all description of the process of comparative analysis touches upon a problem of comparative ethnography which we have not seen raised in methods texts (and were only alerted to by the perceptive comments of one referee responding to Bloor and Fonkert's 'pilot' comparative paper). We refer here to the way in which the attempt to depict similarities and contrasts between communities may itself lead one to under-emphasise the unique features of a setting. Take, for example, the case just mentioned above in which staff were the audience for redefinitional work while planning interventions in their staff meetings. Although this certainly occurred at Camphill it was, as we have said, a much less prominent feature there than at Beeches. Bloor was certainly right to suggest to McKeganey that he draw the reader's attention to the way in which co-workers at Camphill became the target for each other's redefinitions and right to suggest that this was a common feature of instrumental communities, in that it is essential for the collective planning of therapy. Yet by simply noting that this *was* a common feature one inevitably gave the collective planning of interventions at Camphill an unwarranted prominence: both at Camphill and Parkneuk individual co-workers had a lot of autonomy in the determination of their relationships with the individual children and residents in their charge. While in this instance we could alert the reader to the differential salience of collective staff planning, one wonders how often similar distortions have passed from analyst to reader, unnoticed and unnoted, a natural consequence of the comparative method? The comparative method reflexively constructs the 'seeing' of the researcher.

In writing this book we decided against the easy option of passively juxtaposing discrete ethnographies of each setting. But, in merging these descriptions in a comparative treatment of common themes, we have risked losing the unique strength of ethnography – the depiction of a mix of cultural practices in a particular and unique constellation, in a particular and unique context. There is a sense in which comparative ethnography is not ethnography at all. Anthropologists have long been aware of these problems of comparison (Evans-Pritchard, 1960); sociologists using ethnographic methods should be similarly leery.

The participant-observer observed

As Hammersley and Atkinson (1983) have pointed out, all social research (and all social life!) is founded upon participant observation: all researchers are inescapably part of the social world they study. In this last section we examine two aspects of this reflexive relationship as they occurred in our fieldwork. First, we consider the impact on our field relations (and on our data) of the social roles we played in the field settings, not just the roles we chose for ourselves – junior staff member, chauffeur, drinking partner, or whatever – but those thrust upon us by the ascribed statuses of gender, age and ethnicity. And second, we consider the impact on ourselves – our beliefs, behaviour and relationships – of our field relationships.

The three of us are white and male and, at the time of our fieldwork, we were in our twenties and thirties. We have little to say on the racial dimension of field relations. Blacks were absent from some our our settings (such as Parkneuk), in others they were a small minority: our relations with black residents therefore reflected the relations between those residents and other community members, especially the white staff. Three of the study settings were in Scotland, catering for a predominantly Scottish clientele, and Bloor and McKeganey are both English. We judge this to have been of little significance, particularly since in two of the three settings (Parkneuk and the Camphill community) Scottish co-workers were in a minority.

The gender aspect deserves more attention. Despite the undeniable influence which gender exerts on field relations and data collection it is really only with the development of the women's movement that the topic has received more than a cursory discussion. Not surprisingly most recent attention has focused on the role of women in the research process either as researchers, respondents, or both (Easterday et al., 1977; Finch, 1984; Oakley, 1981). We hope to provide an equivalent account of the way in which the researchers' maleness may influence the research process. We should say here that identifying the impact of gender in our work has been (for us) a difficult task. In part, this has to do with the intrinsic difficulties of disentangling gender from a whole host of other biographical and situational factors. In addition, however, there are the difficulties of reflecting on a received status which is both ubiquitous and largely taken for granted. If we concentrate here on those occasions in our fieldwork where gender became particularly prominent it is not because we doubt its impact in the other areas of our work but because of the difficulties we have found in identifying its influence.

In some of our communities gender had a very obvious impact on our research activity. At Faswells, for example, while residents of both sexes mixed socially in the common areas of the ward, dormitories were seen as largely out of bounds for individuals of the opposite sex. While McKeganey could spend time chatting with ease to the males, or playing table tennis with them in their dormitory, he had no equivalent access to the female dormitory and consequently no access to the females' 'world' within this part of the ward.

Even where physical access was not restricted, field relationships with female residents could be problematic. In part, as we shall see, this had to do with local expectations and social taboos; in addition, however, it had to do with the researchers' own fears of being drawn into a situation where accusations of assault from female residents could have resulted. An extract from McKeganey's fieldnotes illustrates this level of concern:

> This afternoon I had taken a group of children along to the main hall for a classical music recital. One of the girls (Clare) was very disturbed, often breaking out in a low moan that wound up into a piercing shriek. It was obvious that someone was going to have to take her out of the hall and Kirsten (co-worker) asked me if I would walk her back to the house. When we arrived the house was empty. Clare flew up to the dormitory and immediately began flinging things around the room. I decided to go up and see what I could do. When I entered the dormitory Clare was stood on the bed resembling nothing so much as a cornered

> animal. She let out a further wail and kicked the bedclothes to the floor. As I moved closer she launched herself at me in a cat-like scratching attack. I could hold her off, but only just. Tired out from the physical exertion, she calmed down. As I got up to leave, though, the whole performance began again. I decided to sit it out, chat to her and wait for one of the other adults to return. Throughout all this I felt distinctly uncomfortable as to how my being alone with a fifteen-year-old girl in her dormitory might be read by the others. Somehow I think Clare was aware of my anxieties and was consciously manipulating me through them.

Although McKeganey did spend time talking to the female residents at Camphill, his contact with them was often underpinned by these sorts of concerns. Similarly, Bloor (who slept in the residents' quarters at Ashley) was so concerned about one girl's (joking?) wish to see what he looked like when asleep that he mentioned the matter to the staff member on overnight duty before he went to bed, covering himself (he hoped) against any future suspicion. Oddly enough, there were no comparable fears and uncertainties about individual contacts with male residents, although homosexual activities were known to occur amongst residents in at least two of the communities.

In some of our communities the researchers were involved in group discussions on the topic of the attraction that residents, male as well as female, felt for the researcher, and the reciprocal attraction the researcher felt for individual residents. (In one community the researcher was surprised to learn subsequently that staff had rather anticipated events by describing him to residents as an attractive young sociologist.) These discussions were sometimes stressful to participate in but on occasion allowed the air to be cleared sufficiently for good and frank individual field relationships between the researcher and female residents to develop.

It is extremely difficult to know how determining these concerns of gender and sexuality were within the fieldwork context. Bloor, for example, although experiencing these concerns in relation to contacts with female residents in their bedrooms and on outings (which might be construed as dating) still felt able to strike up naturalistic and productive individual relationships with female residents outside of these areas providing, that is, he adopted a viable marginal role. At the outset of his fieldwork at Ashley, Bloor noted that:

> I think it might be quite difficult to chat naturally to the girls: they seem to be used only to relationships with men of a sexual, or sexually bantering, kind. They seem to choose only female staff as their confidantes.

Yet some months later, a female staff member watched slightly enviously as Bloor (back for another fortnight's fieldwork) was surrounded by excited, hugging female residents. She commented 'I know who you are – you're the favourite uncle'. McKeganey gravitated into a similar 'favourite uncle' role at the Camphill community. But not everyone has or wants to have a 'favourite uncle' in their social network. Nor does everyone wish to have their memory of a favourite uncle rekindled by the researcher's role playing. McKeganey recorded the following discussion during one of the large group meetings at Faswells at which his participation in the small groups was being decided upon:

> EILEEN (resident): I don't want Neil to come into my group because I'll feel inhibited.
> STEVE (nurse): Would you feel inhibited with a tape recorder?
> EILEEN: I don't want either.
> GAIL (nurse): Can you say why?
> EILEEN: Because Neil reminds me of my uncle who I liked. He looked like Neil and he did something in scientific research.
> GAIL: Do you have some fantasy, Eileen, about how your relationship with Neil would develop if he came into the group?
> EILEEN: I just feel that I don't want people to get close to me. When they do I always end up making demands on them and they end up not liking me.

Throughout this fieldwork McKeganey did not feel able to find an equivalent social role to Bloor's 'favourite uncle' and never really felt able, in his own mind, to resolve satisfactorily his concerns about the level and quality of his contact with female residents.

It is, of course, an open question whether negotiating such a role is equivalent to minimising the impact of gender itself. It is possible that gender continued to have an impact, though one we were unaware of, even on those occasions when our anxieties about contacts with female residents were allayed.

Gender was not, however, experienced simply as an obstacle to be overcome in this research. Indeed, in our contacts with male residents we were often able to trade off the fact of our maleness in building relationships with them. Bloor was able to occupy the role of drinking partner with some of the male residents in his communities, and McKeganey spent a good deal of time playing table tennis at Faswells and Ravenscroft – an activity that was almost exclusively male in both communities. Yet while the fact of our maleness may have facilitated these relationships it might also have set limits to them. There may have been some things, for example, which male residents held from us precisely because we were also males.

On the whole, our relationships with staff were collegial. At Beeches, for example, Bloor would frequently visit the pub with a male residential staff member. At Ashley the only staff member resident in the house was a female student volunteer; she and Bloor were often in each other's company in the house, but only went to the pub with others – to have done otherwise would have been tantamount to dating.

Obviously the question of how much of an impact gender has had on our work is not one we can answer definitively. We cannot, for example, suggest ways in which our accounts would have differed had our gender been different. Nevertheless, it seems unlikely that our description of therapeutic work would have been greatly different from that which we have provided in this book. Certainly we did not have the impression that, for example, male and female residents and staff members saw therapeutic work in these settings in massively different terms.

We have said very little so far on the question of age, which, like gender, is a designation that often carries with it a whole host of associated meanings. In four of our communities (Parkneuk, Camphill, Ashley and Beeches) there was an age difference between the researchers and the residents that was sometimes transcendable and sometimes a potential barrier to close field relations. One remedy for such difficulties lay in establishing naturalistic field relations which acknowledged and incorporated that age difference. Such a remedy mirrors the position adopted by many of the staff in their relations with adolescents: recall Len's behaviour while watching *Match of the Day* at Beeches (instanced in Chapter 3) – he was not being 'one of the boys' but was simply reacting to Harry, Kevin and Terry in a naturalistic, relaxed, friendly and rather father-like way. Presumably another possible remedy would have been to make the age difference an explicit focus of therapeutic work in the same way that sexual attractiveness on occasion was.

For the most part, staff in communities were of a similar age and background to the researchers – many even had the same record collections!

Whilst age, gender and ethnicity are all ascribed statuses, carrying with them advantages and disadvantages for fieldwork relations, it would be a mistake to view them as wholly determining. More correctly, a fieldworker's ascribed statuses represent areas of participation, areas where the fieldworker trades on his or her gender, age or ethnicity with the object of establishing naturalistic field relations – relations, that is, in which it is the researcher's person, rather than their status, which is more prominent. In some situations, of course, it may simply not be possible, however personable the researcher is, to overcome these statuses – one imagines, for example, that it would be very difficult for a black individual to sustain naturalistic field relations in a Ku Klux Klan gathering.

We turn now from the specific issue of ascribed statuses in fieldwork relationships to the wider topic of the negotiation of the participant observer's 'participation' in the fieldwork setting. Again we shall see these negotiations as occurring within a network of expectations and shall examine the limitations and advantages of the particular roles we adopted and were constrained to adopt.

On entering any setting the researcher is likely to find members with existing views of the researcher's role, and indeed members who act toward the researcher on the basis of these views. Two early fieldnotes:

> Talking in OT to Betty ... She said she's been a bit non-plussed by my behaviour. When my arrival had been spoken of in the group, she'd pictured a much more clinical approach ('all these interviews and tests, and filling out cards, and that').

> Lisa ... reminisced about previous occasions when inadequate specificity (of procedures) had led to confusion and worse: one resident had taken too literally the fire drill instruction to make for the nearest exit and had jumped through the first floor window. Lisa suggested this incident was something I might like to use to spice up my write-up. She's used it several times in presentations on the work of the house. Lisa is still very much aware of my presence as a researcher.

That there are no rules of fieldwork conduct for the researcher to apply, template-like, to relations with respondents is an opportunity as well as a problem (Cunningham-Burley, 1987), and the participant observer role embraces a spectrum of degrees of engagement. In our fieldwork we found ourselves close to the 'most engaged' end of this spectrum. There are now numerous examples of sociological studies where the fieldworker is simultaneously researcher and member (we follow Emerson, 1981, in distinguishing these 'member-researcher' studies from covert fieldwork, because the research effort is explicitly identified). In fact, one of the attractions of therapeutic communities as research locales is the unique opportunity they present for medical sociologists to gather data on the practice of therapeutic work as a participant. Various advantages can accrue from this particular kind of participation: relative to a less engaged approach, it may be easier to gain an understanding of particular kinds of members' activities; participation may be a test of the adequacy of one's understanding; and participation is also a source of gratification.

Projects which seek to know people's minds demand particular methods (Psathas, 1968), and participation in staff work was an appropriate method for a project which conceived of therapeutic work as an act of cognition – a sometimes silent gaze, a momentary glance. From the standpoint of the German hermeneutic philosophers, knowledge of a culture is only possible by the immersion of the observer in a 'form of life'. We do not argue, as some researchers would, that this kind of knowledge is only accessible to the member-researcher who actually performs the activities, as opposed to the non-member who empathetically observes. But we do take it to be self-evident that such access is easier for the member-researcher: immersion proceeds faster with direct involvement.

To get to know a form of life is to be able to find one's way about in it, to be able to sustain encounters with others in the research setting (Giddens, 1976, p. 149). Being able to perform as a staff member ('passing': Douglas, 1976, pp. 123–4) may not always be an adequate test of knowledge of therapeutic work: in some settings others (staff and residents) may tolerate quite wide variations in staff performance, and in other settings staff work may be more guided by external regulation. Nevertheless, in some communities acceptance by others of the researcher's performance as that of a staff member may be relevant to judging the adequacy of the researcher's understanding.

The importance of having a gratifying sense of one's usefulness in the research setting need not be laboured to anyone who has experienced the discomforts of extreme marginality:

> Robert asked me if I'll be coming to do fieldwork much longer. The hope that lies behind the question is that I'll be able to help out in the [horticultural] field with the spring planting – a busy time. One of the things that makes fieldwork so pleasant is the knowledge that my help with the work is needed and appreciated.

Enumeration of the advantages of the member-researcher role should not be read as implying that such roles are always freely chosen. One's fieldwork role is always a matter of on-going negotiation in the research setting, and, as we have repeatedly stated, there is a Utopian strain in therapeutic community practice. The very processes that so successfully induct and enthuse incoming residents and new staff are also a snare for the incoming researcher. Even if the researcher is immune to this tide of Utopian enthusiasm, he or she may find it an uncomfortable and occasionally untenable position to be marginal in a role that is by turns cosily domestic and highly emotional. We chose our member-researcher roles but we could well have found that negotiations would have led us toward similar positions in any case: several times we heard staff and residents express the view that the research role we adopted was probably the only viable way to research their communities.

The disadvantages of the member-researcher role are obvious: first, the temptation to 'go native', abandon the researcher role and submerge ourselves in the staff projects; and second, the problem of bias.

Self-evidently, we did not go native, though there were occasions when writing our fieldnotes seemed a tiresome irrelevance. Rereading our fieldnotes, we actually encounter something of a puzzle. Our notes sometimes reveal such a degree of engagement with events in the community that it is rather difficult to explain how we summoned or retained the necessary reflectivity to write them at all. For example, Bloor's remarks on the strength of his feelings after he led the day hospital 'fantasy' (one person describes a fantasy journey while the rest of the encounter group lie down, close their eyes, and try to visualise it):

> I have heard staff especially (but also occasionally patients) refer to their concern for the group. Thus, I remember Oliver once

> called the group his 'family'. I couldn't follow this . . . In fact I doubted the sincerity of those who expressed themselves in this way. But today I realised that I now felt the same way. Nancy (patient) was speaking of her good feelings when, on a previous occasion, she had taken the fantasy and watched protectively over the huddle of forms as she spoke. I realised that I had felt the same as I led the fantasy. I spoke about my strong feelings about the group and expressing the thought strengthened it further, till I actually felt tears pricking my eyes.

We offer three comments on the rather paradoxical existence of such fieldnotes – fieldnotes which communicate our engagement in the setting but, by the very fact of being noted, imply a measure of detached reflectivity. In the first place, neither the researcher nor the member roles are roles in the Lintonian sense of the term. Rather, following Bates (1956) we see various sets of normative prescriptions associated with each social position. Just as it was possible for Len, playing football, to be a member of staff and father-like, so also it was possible for the fieldworker to entertain a number of different (and even incipiently contradictory) normative prescriptions within the same social position.

In the second place, we were never full-time participants in any of the settings. Fonkert was not residential during the concept house study, McKeganey and Bloor were only in part-time attendance at the Camphill community and the day hospital. Bloor conducted his fieldwork at the halfway houses on a two-weeks-on-two-weeks-off residential basis and so on: periodic departure from the settings provided occasions for reflection.

In the third place, engagement was called forth most insistently in those communities using reality-confronting techniques, but these techniques also promote reflectivity. The self-same processes that were engaging the researcher in the settings were inculcating habits of reflection and observation. Most communities also employ particular organisational techniques, such as staff review groups, to promote such reflectivity. As Pollner and Emerson (1983, p. 247n.) have noted, there are clear resemblances between the ways in which researchers manage field relations and the practices of other professionals, such as psychotherapists, who strive simultaneously to establish both rapport and distance. In our research the culture of the setting may have promoted a reflectivity which is lost in most cultures when one accedes to membership.

In respect of the bias issue, it is true that all research methods – experimental methods included – have their impact on the phenomenon under study, so this need be no cause for excessive concern. Nevertheless, we can identify four ways in which our participation may have had an impact on the phenomena being studied and the data being collected: first, through the researchers' contributions (positive or negative) to practice; second, through the loss of information that is concealed from the staff gaze – the loss of the residents' perspective; third, through the requirement to regulate one's contacts with residents in a manner that would be approved by the staff; and fourth, through the unknown (and largely unknowable) impact of variations in the researchers' personalities.

With respect to the researchers' contributions to staff practice we judge this to have occurred not primarily through the 'Hawthorne effect' of people being spurred to action as a result of being observed but rather through the fact of the researcher's presence enlarging the staff group and so increasing the possibilities for therapeutic work. Consider, for example, the responses of two staff members at Ashley to Bloor's question about whether his presence had led staff into being more 'interventionist':

> Frank considered this quite carefully . . . he had certainly been aware of my presence during the pilot period and he recollected that there had been some initial disquiet among staff about my presence (largely centring around an uncertainty about how far I would be an active participant in the community). However, this had quite rapidly disappeared as far as he was concerned. He thought it was unlikely that staff would feel pressured into more interventionist behaviour by my presence for two main reasons: firstly, staff behaviour was practised and repetitive – over time staff would tend to gravitate back to their routine behaviour regardless of being observed. Secondly, there is a regular procession of social work students through the house and staff are used to carrying out their jobs in front of such observers. In this respect Frank thought my presence was less disruptive than the social work students, in whose presence he sometimes felt constrained to spell out the thinking behind his actions in much more detail than would be necessary with staff members or myself.

Frank had considered the question from the standpoint of

'Hawthorne effects', but Neil appeared to consider it from the standpoint of group dynamics:

> I asked Neil if he thought he was more interventionist when I was around. Yes, he thought so. It was perhaps because, when there were other staff there, then there was an opportunity to do more work. Was this the case with social work students? Oh no, but I'd been around the house such a long time now.

One of the Parkneuk co-workers made a similar point: things were 'different' at the community on the days that Bloor was there because his presence was an 'additional factor' in the relationships at Parkneuk. Where therapeutic work is the object of the study, and where these community relationships are a medium of therapeutic work, then the participant observer's activity is clearly an important component in the reflexive constitution of therapy.

This is not simply an issue that surfaces for researchers who participate as staff members. When Bloor was conducting research at the day hospital his interest in the relationship of the patient culture to the formal treatment programme led him to spend all his time initially with the day hospital patients. At the end of his research, he was mortified to be told by a patient that the patients always seemed a more cohesive group when Bloor was around: by chatting to all the patients impartially Bloor had inhibited cliquey exclusiveness and social isolation. The researcher had unwittingly taken a leading role in shaping the patient culture he intended to study.

To regard the adoption of a member-researcher role within the staff group as entailing the loss of the residents' perspective is an oversimplification. There was no residents' counter-culture opposed to the staff project and providing interpretations competitive with staff redefinitions (see Chapter 5). Staff redefinitions were contested on occasion, but more normally by individuals than by a group. On such occasions staff often won support for their contested viewpoint from other residents. There was no residents' perspective, but there was a residents' 'backstage', with criticism of staff, horse-play, in-jokes, shared confidences, and tacit agreements – a world of pubs and parties and kitchen gossip, a world that is only glimpsed by the researcher who participates in the community as a staff member. When Bloor became a member of the staff group at the day hospital he was surprised and uncomfortable about the volume of insider knowledge to which he had unwittingly become a party by his previous membership of the patient group, knowledge that he realised was largely hidden from the staff. However, ours is a study of therapeutic work, it is not a study of the residents' world.

A third and related aspect of the bias issue concerns the way in which the member-researcher's field relationships with residents may be constrained by the need to negotiate those relationships within approved staff guidelines. Consider, for example a difficulty McKeganey faced at one point in his fieldwork. He had struck up a fairly close relationship with one of the female residents – a relationship which, had the individual concerned been of the same sex as the researcher, one would have categorised as that of 'key informant' (Whyte, 1955). The fact that the resident was not of the same sex raised a whole host of alternative interpretations of the relationship, not all of which were particularly positive. Indeed, during the fieldwork McKeganey himself came to question the relationship. When the girl's name came up in staff meetings McKeganey was wary of expressing a contrary opinion to that held by staff lest they view his response as indicating his having too close a relationship with the girl to form an independent opinion.

It was not that staff expected us as researchers to have the *same* relationships with residents that they themselves had. Rather, in the above instance, staff would have expected that McKeganey's relationship would be openly discussed – become a topic for therapeutic work – so that any elements which the staff might term projection or transference could be examined and responded to. Nevertheless, the requirement to make such a close fieldwork relationship a topic for group discussion was in itself a form of constraint. In effect, McKeganey faced a dilemma in either facing staff disapproval of a 'covert' key informant relationship which might be interpreted as destructive 'pairing', or in assenting to the constraint of making this relationship open to discussion and possible transmutation (several of the fieldwork relationships we formed with residents were discussed in this manner). In the end, McKeganey resolved to reduce his contact.

Staff, not researchers, carry the final responsibility for resident welfare and it is entirely appropriate that bounds should be put on the field relations of researchers where these touch on resident treatment. We endorse the necessity for such constraints and raise the matter here simply to emphasise that they *are* constraints.

While we would accept that our choice of working in the role of staff members has influenced our data collection, and therefore our descriptions of these settings, we are much less clear as to the influence which our individual personalities or personas may have had on our work. The impact of personality within the research context is, like gender, extremely difficult to assess, not least because of the difficulties of knowing what the term refers to. Like many terms from psychology and sociology 'personality' has found its way into popular discourse where its meaning is no longer clear cut. It is largely in the sense of its everyday usage that we refer to the term here – that is, as a gloss for a whole host of individual biographical features, for example, temperament, likes, dislikes, behavioural style, mode of dress. It is self-evident, to us if not to the reader, that each of the researchers is very different in some if not all these respects. It would be comforting in scientific terms to assume that none of these things has had a determining impact on our research activity. We cannot, however, be quite so confident, since on occasion staff and residents themselves drew attention to this impact. At the end of fieldwork in one of the settings, staff commented to McKeganey, for example, that although they had initially had some reservations about the prospect of being observed they had actually enjoyed the experience. One of the nurses drew attention to McKeganey's personal style, commenting that this was one aspect which had made the reality of being researched less daunting than the prospect:

> You could have come in here and said – I'm Dr. McKeganey and I'll be studying your work – but you didn't. You were just yourself and I know that made me feel a lot easier and I think it made the residents feel a lot easier as well.

In one of the other settings McKeganey was consciously aware of limiting his contacts with one particular resident – a large, aggressive-looking individual who, it seemed to McKeganey, was in a permanent state of barely suppressed rage. The fact that McKeganey felt more comfortable with certain residents and indeed certain staff than others, did then, have an impact on the sorts of field relations he sustained.

It is undeniable that each of the researchers felt more comfortable in some situations than others, and with some individuals more than others. Yet it would be misleading to suggest that our own personal affinities remained unchanged across the settings in which we were collecting data. Bloor, for example, had the feeling of acting in a different way across the different settings in which he was collecting data. He also, crucially, had the sense of becoming close to some individuals in the day hospital to whom he guessed he would not have been attracted had he met them under different circumstances.

It seems to us, then, that our individual personalities and personal styles have influenced our field relations and indeed been influenced in turn by those relations. However, the extent to which these factors have influenced our description of the various settings is an unanswerable question. Indeed, one could only come to an understanding of these things by comparing the accounts of two researchers of quite different temperaments and personal styles working in the same setting, at the same time, and researching the same topic.

We should add one rider to these speculations: in scientific discourse, indeed in most areas of our lives, we generally do not suppose that the information we are provided with is reducible to the personality of the individual concerned. Rightly or wrongly we ordinarily assume that if personality comes into it at all it does so in only a limited way. Malinowski appears to have been much irritated by his native informants, but it is not suggested that the publication of his fieldwork diaries revealing his irritation seriously undermines his analysis.

Finally, we turn to the question of the impact which this research has had on us – as individuals. At times during this research we cried, shook with anger, creased with laughter, and felt the deepest fellowship with community members. In cthnography this engagement with one's subject must co-exist with the more or less normal performance of domestic and academic relationships, sometimes with very odd results. Barker (1984) reported that her spouse was much surprised when he happened to witness one of her conversations with her Moonie subjects – she seemed quite a different person from her normal self. Our spouses sometimes had similarly surprising encounters:

> My farewell party . . . I was presented with a cigarette lighter to which all the patients and staff had contributed (this is stranger than it seems . . . no-one had previously been given a gift on leaving. . .) The party was a very emotional occasion with everyone saying (repeatedly in some instances) how fond they were of me and what a nice person I was. My wife was quite nonplussed . . . when I returned the following afternoon to collect my record-player my host asked me if I'd be best man at his wedding.

But this spouse was not comparing the researcher persona with an inviolate domestic persona, because the domestic persona was also somewhat changed. In part, this was due to the importation of the stresses and strains of fieldwork into domestic life – recurrent tiredness, the need to find the time to write up fieldnotes *and* have some domestic and social life, and so on. (Parenthetically, we believe we discovered the sovereign remedy for this – the conduct of fieldwork in short residential blocks, interspersed by equivalent home visits. This was Bloor's modus operandi on his last study – Ashley and Beeches. Under these circumstances, loyalties are no longer stretched, or commitments cross-cut: domestic life becomes a joyous relief and a haven for detachment.) In part also, changes in domestic persona were the result of a process of reality construction. Residents were expected to leave the treatment setting and apply to their outside relationships their new-learned understandings, skills and patterns of relationship. The member-researcher is similarly influenced. Friends were surprised to get an uncharacteristic phone call from one researcher asking them to postpone at the last minute an evening visit, because (he explained) researcher and spouse were in the middle of their monthly row! 'Honest relations' were to the fore.

As well as being influenced by the process of gaining membership of these settings we have also been affected by the process of leaving. As in so many areas of our lives the depth of our attachment to friends, colleagues, family, etc. is often only realised at the point where these contacts are coming to an end. It would be overly dramatic to suggest that we experienced separation anxieties on withdrawing from the field; nevertheless, the speed with which the transition from insider to outsider often occurred was something we had to cope with. McKeganey attempted to ease his withdrawal from the field by returning to one community on a weekly basis – it was a strategy that had its own difficulties:

> Going back one day a week seems much more difficult than I ever imagined it would be. I want to clear this up in my own mind and maybe writing this fieldnote will help. I guess the main difficulty is simply not knowing where I stand in relation to so much. In a way one of the most puzzling things is the simplicity in the children's emotions towards me. Each Saturday they greet me as a long lost friend and I know that many look forward to my visits. Alongside this, though, there is a mass of uncertainty and misunderstanding. I think one thing sparked off these

> feelings. This evening, I was in one of the dormitories helping one of the co-workers cut a child's nails. Another boy came in and sat on my knee. In fun I cut a lock off his hair and replaced it with a piece of my own. I then held the two pieces together and showed him the difference in colour – he laughed. Later the dormitory parent came in and demanded to know who had cut the boy's hair. I said nothing though I could tell he was pretty cross ... The whole thing got out of hand. I can't help feeling that if I had been living there and this happened we could have seen it as a bit of fun. Coming one day a week makes this so different ... Sometimes I feel a stranger in the house. But yet not really a stranger, as I have known, lived and worked with most of the adults and kids. The change from day to night brings a change in how I feel about being in the house. It's as if in darkness I am like a guest who has stayed too long. I think I should speak to the houseparent about not coming any more on a regular basis.

By their very nature therapeutic communities are highly dynamic environments to live and work within. While this accounts for much of their appeal it is also the very thing which makes returning as a visitor such a disheartening experience. Yet even in this we have found some variability between our communities. We noted in Chapter 2 that Parkneuk community resonated with a warmth and an openness that seemed to persist irrespective of changes in personnel. This study began with Parkneuk so perhaps it is appropriate that returning to this community should have been so easy.

In spite of the feelings of acute marginality often surrounding our immediate departure it is probably just as well that the impact of having lived and worked in these settings has been softened over time both by new experiences and the reassertion of old habits. Even the most cathartic of our fieldwork experiences are now covered by a warm patina of remembrance. But our lives have been touched and changed by our experiences. Were we anthropologists then therapeutic communities would be our 'tribe'. And we acknowledge that fact with gratitude. To paraphrase our favourite anthropologist (Geertz, 1973), if our scientific imagination has been powerful enough to put readers in touch with the lives of these strangers in their communities, then the effort of writing this book has been (almost) worthwhile.

Bibliography

Apte, R. (1966), 'The transitional hostel in the rehabilitation of the mentally ill', in G. McLachlan (ed.), *Problems and Progress in Medical Care*, London, Nuffield Provincial Hospitals Trust.

Armstrong, D. (1983), *Political Anatomy of the Body: Medical Knowledge in Britain in the Twentieth Century*, Cambridge, Cambridge University Press.

Auden, W. H., (1930), *The English Auden: poems, essays and dramatic writings 1927–1939*, London, Faber & Faber. And *Collected Poems*, Mendelson, E. (ed.), New York, Random House.

Bachrach, P. and Baratz, H. (1962), 'The two faces of power', *American Political Science Review*, vol. 56, pp. 121–35.

Barker, E. (1984), *The Making of a Moonie: Choice or Brainwashing?,* Oxford, Blackwell.

Barnes, M. and Berke, J. (1973), *Mary Barnes, Two Accounts of a Journey through Madness*, Harmondsworth, Penguin.

Barratt, B. (1978), 'The therapeutic community today in the penal services', paper given at the Anglo-Dutch Workshop on Therapeutic Communities, Windsor.

Barton, R. (1959), *Institutional Neurosis*, Bristol, Wright.

Basaglia, F. (1981), 'Breaking the circle of control' in D. Ingleby (ed.), *Critical Psychiatry*, Harmondsworth, Penguin.

Bates, F. (1956), 'Position, role and status: a reformulation', *Social Forces*, vol. 34, pp. 313–21.

Bazeley, E. (1928), *Homer Lane and the Little Commonwealth*, London, Allen & Unwin.

Beknap, I. (1956), *Human Problems of a State Mental Hospital*, New York, McGraw-Hill.

Berger, P. and Luckmann, T. (1967), *The Social Construction of Reality*, Harmondsworth, Allen Lane.

Berke, J. (1980), 'Therapeutic community models: II, Kingsley Hall (UK)', in E. Jansen (ed.), *The Therapeutic Community*, London, Croom Helm.

Blake, R. (1977), 'ATC prospects', *Bulletin of the Association of Therapeutic Communities*, no. 22, pp. 15–16.

Bloor, M. (1976), 'Professional autonomy and client exclusion, a study in

ENT clinics', in M. Wadsworth and D. Robinson (eds), *Studies in Everyday Medical Life*, London, Martin Robertson.

Bloor, M. (1978), 'On the analysis of observational data: a discussion of the worth and uses of inductive techniques and respondent validation', *Sociology*, vol. 12, pp. 545–52.

Bloor, M. (1980a), 'The relationships between informal patient interaction and the formal treatment programme in a psychiatric day hospital using therapeutic community treatment methods', Institute of Medical Sociology Occasional Paper, no. 4, University of Aberdeen.

Bloor, M. (1980b), 'The nature of therapeutic work in therapeutic communities: some preliminary findings', *International Journal of Therapeutic Communities*, vol. 1, pp. 180–91.

Bloor, M. (1981), 'Therapeutic paradox – the relationship between the patient culture and the formal treatment programme in a therapeutic community', *British Journal of Medical Psychology*, vol. 54, pp. 359–69.

Bloor, M. (1984), 'A comparison of two contrasting halfway houses organised as therapeutic communities', Institute of Medical Sociology Occasional Paper, no. 6, University of Aberdeen.

Bloor, M. (1986a), 'Problems of therapeutic community practice in two halfway houses for adolescents', *Journal of Adolescence*, vol. 9, pp. 29–48.

Bloor, M. (1986b), 'Contrasting therapeutic community practices in two halfway houses for disturbed adolescents', *International Journal of Therapeutic Communities*, vol. 7, pp. 5–24.

Bloor, M. (1986c), 'Social control in the therapeutic community: re-examination of a critical case', *Sociology of Health and Illness*, vol. 8, pp. 305–24.

Bloor, M. (1986d), 'Cleaning up the therapeutic community', *New Society*, 31 January, pp. 185–6.

Bloor, M. and Fonkert, J. D. (1982), 'Reality construction, reality exploration, and treatment in two therapeutic communities', *Sociology of Health and Illness*, vol. 4, pp. 125–140.

Bloor, M. and Harris, R. (1984), 'Alienation and medical care, a contribution to the Illich/Navarro dispute', unpublished MS.

Bloor, M. and McKeganey, N. (1986), 'Conceptions of therapeutic work in therapeutic communities', *International Journal of Sociology and Social Policy*, vol. 6, 68–79.

Boulay, J. du and Williams, R. (1987) 'To see ourselves: images of the fieldworker in Scotland and Greece with some reflections upon fieldwork', in McKeganey, N. and Cunningham-Burley, S. (eds), *Enter the Sociologist: Reflections on the Practice of Sociology*, Aldershot, Gower.

Boyle, J. (1977), *A Sense of Freedom*, London, Pan.

Braginsky, B., Braginsky, D. and Ring, K. (1969), *Methods of Madness – the Mental Hospital as a Last Resort*, New York, Holt, Rinehart, and Winston.

Bremer, I., Fonkert, J. D., Korswagen, K., Kouwershoven, H., van Procijen, A., Samwel, T., Veldkamp, D., van Westing, J. and Maso, I. (1977), 'Sociologische dieple-interviews met verslavings-therapeuten',

Fenomenologisch-Sociologisch Onderzoek II, Leiden, Sociologisch Instituut.
Caudill, W. (1958), *The Psychiatric Hospital as a Small Society*, Cambridge, Harvard University Press.
Clark, D. (1965), 'The therapeutic community: concept, practice, and future', *British Journal of Psychiatry*, vol. 111, pp. 947–54.
Clark, D. (1977), 'The therapeutic community', *British Journal of Psychiatry*, vol. 131, pp. 553–64.
Clarke, B. (1974), *Enough room for joy: Jean Vanier's L'Arche a message for our time*, London, Longman & Todd.
Cooley, C. (1983), *Human Nature and Social Order*, London, Transaction. (original edition, 1902)
Cooper, D. (1967), *Psychiatry and Anti-Psychiatry*, London, Tavistock.
Coser, L. (1974), *Greedy Institutions*, New York, Free Press.
Croall, J. (1983), *Neill of Summerhill, the Permanent Rebel*, London, Routledge & Kegan Paul.
Cunningham-Burley, S. (1987), 'The data fix' in McKeganey, N. and Cunningham-Burley, S. (eds), *Enter the Sociologist: Reflections of the Practice of Sociology*, Aldershot, Gower.
Dalley, G. (1983), 'Ideologies of care: a feminist contribution to the debate', *Critical Social Policy*, no. 19, pp. 72–81.
Dockar-Drysdale, B. (1968), *Therapy in Child Care*, London, Longmans.
Douglas, Jack B. (1976), *Investigative Social Research: Individual and Team Research*, Beverley Hills, Sage.
Easterday, L., Papademas, D., Schoor, L. and Valentine, C. (1977), 'The making of a female researcher', *Urban Life*, vol. 6, pp. 333–48.
Emerson, R. (1981), 'Obervational fieldwork', *Annual Review of Sociology*, vol. 7, pp. 351–78.
Evans-Pritchard, E. (1960), Introduction to R. Hertz, *Death and the Right Hand*, London, Cohen & West.
Finch, J. (1984), 'It's great to have someone to talk to: ethics and politics of interviewing women', in C. Bell and H. Roberts (eds), *Social Researching: Politics, Problems and Practice*, London, Routledge & Kegan Paul.
Fisher, L. (1976), 'Dropping remarks and the Barbadian audience', *American Ethnologist*, vol. 13, pp. 227–42.
Fletcher, C. (1974), *Beneath the Surface, an Account of Three Styles of Sociological Research*, London, Routledge & Kegan Paul.
Fonkert, J. D. (1978), 'Reality construction in a therapeutic community for ex-drug-addicts', doctoral dissertation, The Hague.
Foucault, M. (1973), *The Birth of the Clinic*, (trans. A. M. Sheridan), London, Tavistock.
Foucault, M. (1980), 'The eye of power' in M. Foucault, *Power/Knowledge*, (C. Gordon ed.), London, Harvester.
Frye, N. (1967), 'Literary Utopias', in F. Manuel (ed.), *Utopias and Utopian Thought*, Boston, Beacon.
Gadamer, H. (1976), *Philosophical Hermeneutics*, Berkeley, University of California Press.
Garfinkel, H. (1967), *Studies in Ethnomethodology*, Englewood Cliffs, N.J., Prentice-Hall.

Gauthier, P. (1980), 'Psycho-education as a re-education model, theoretical foundations and practical implications', in E. Jansen (ed.), *The Therapeutic Community*, London, Croom Helm.

Geertz, C. (1973), 'Thick description: toward an interpretative theory of culture', in C. Geertz, *The Interpretation of Cultures: Selected Essays*, New York, Basic Books.

Gibbon, L. G. (1971), *Sunset Song*, London, Longmans.

Giddens, A. (1976), *New Rules of Sociological Method, a Positive Critique of Interpretative Methodologies*, London, Hutchinson.

Goffman, E. (1959), *Presentation of Self in Everyday Life*, New York, Doubleday-Anchor.

Goffman, E. (1968), *Asylums*, Harmondsworth, Penguin.

Good, B. and Good, M. (1980). 'The meaning of symptoms: a cultural hermeneutic model for clinical practice' in L. Eisenberg and A. Kleinman (eds), *The Relevance of Social Science for Medicine*, Dordrecht, D. Reidel.

Good, B., Herrera, H., Good, H. and Cooper, J. (1985), 'Reflexivity, counter-transference, and clinical ethnography: a case from a psychiatric cultural consultation clinic', in R. Hahn and A. Gaines (eds), *Physicians of Western Medicine*, Dordrecht, D. Reidel.

Gould, L., Walker, A., Crane, L. and Lidz, C. (1974), *Connections: Notes from the Heroin World*, New Haven, Yale University Press.

Haddon, B. (1979), 'Political implications of therapeutic communities' in R. Hinshelwood and N. Manning (eds), *Therapeutic Communities: Reflections and Progress*, London, Routledge & Kegan Paul.

Hammersley, M. and Atkinson, P. (1983), *Ethnography: Principles in Practice*, London, Tavistock.

Herzlich, C. (1976), 'Therapeutic community and psychiatry in the community: a comparative study of the French and Anglo-Saxon literatures', in M. Sokolowsha, J. Holanka and A. Ostravska (eds), *Health, Medicine, Society*, New York, D. Reidel.

Hester, S. (1981), 'Two tensions in ethnomethodology and conversational analyses', *Sociology*, vol. 15, pp. 1–15.

Hoffman, H. (1980), 'The halfway house as a therapeutic community: a useful model of a burdensome myth', in E. Jansen (ed.), *The Therapeutic Community*, London, Croom Helm.

Hoffman, I. and Singer, P. (1977), 'The incompatibility of the medical model and the therapeutic community', *Social Science and Medicine*, vol. 11, pp. 425–31.

Illich, I. (1975), *Medical Nemesis*, London, Calder & Boyars.

Illich, I. (1978), *Limits to Medicine*, Harmondsworth, Penguin.

Illsley, R. (1980), *Professional or Public Health*, London, Nuffield Provincial Hospitals Trust.

Janov, A. (1973), *The Primal Scream*, London, Abacus.

Jansen, E. (1970), 'The role of the halfway house in community mental health programs in the United Kingdom and America', *American Journal of Psychiatry*, vol. 126, pp. 1498–1504.

Jansen, E. (1979), Director's report in *Richmond Fellowship Report 1977–1978*, London, Richmond Fellowship.

Jansen E. (1980), Editor's discussion in E. Jansen (ed.), *The Therapeutic*

Community, London, Croom Helm.
Jansen, E. (1984), *Silver Jubilee Report*, London, Richmond Fellowship.
Jones, M. (1952), *Social Psychiatry*, London, Tavistock.
Jones, M. (1962), *Social Psychiatry in the Community*, Springfield, Charles Thomas.
Jones, M. (1968), *Beyond the Therapeutic Community*, New Haven, Yale University Press.
Jones, M. (1982), *The Process of Change*, London, Routledge & Kegan Paul.
Kanter, R. (1972), *Commitment and Community: Communes and Utopias in Sociological Perspective*, Cambridge, Harvard University Press.
Kennard, D. (1983), *An Introduction to Therapeutic Communities*, London, Routledge & Kegan Paul.
Kennard, D. and Clemmey, R. (1976), 'Psychiatric patients as seen by self and others: an explanation of change in a therapeutic community setting', *British Journal of Medical Psychology*, vol. 43, pp. 35–53.
Kennard, D., Clemmey, R. and Manderbrote, B. (1977), 'Aspects of outcome in a therapeutic community setting – how patients are seen by themselves and others', *British Journal of Psychiatry*, vol. 130, pp. 475–80.
Kesey, K. (1962), *One Flew Over the Cuckoo's Nest*, New York, Victory Press.
King, L. (1954), 'What is disease?', *Philosophy of Science*, vol. 21, pp. 193–200.
Kleinman, A. (1980), *Patients and Healers in the Context of Culture*, Berkeley, University of California Press.
Konig, K. (1965), 'The three essentials of Camphill', *Cresset*, vol. 11, pp. 143–54.
Konig, K. (1975), 'Meaning and value of curative education and curative work', *Camphill Village Trust News*, Spring, pp. 1–2.
Laing, R. D. (1960), *The Divided Self*, London, Tavistock.
Laing, R. D. (1967), *The Politics of Experience and the Bird of Paradise*, Harmondsworth, Penguin.
Laing, R. D., Esterson, A. and Cooper, D. (1965), 'Results of family-oriented therapy with hospitalised schizophrenics', *British Medical Journal*, II, pp. 1462–5.
Leach, J. and Wing, J. (1980), *Helping Destitute Men*, London, Tavistock.
Letemendia, F., Harris, A. and Williams, P. (1967), 'The clinical effect on a population of chronic schizophrenic patients of administrative changes in hospital', *British Journal of Psychiatry*, vol. 113, pp. 959–71.
Lukes, S. (1974), *Power, a Radical View*, London, Macmillan.
McKeganey, N. (1982), 'The social organisation of everyday therapeutic work in a Camphill Rudolf Steiner therapeutic community', Unpublished PhD thesis, University of Aberdeen.
McKeganey, N. (1983), 'The social organisation of everyday therapeutic work – making the backstage visible', *International Journal of Therapeutic Communities*, vol. 4, pp. 13–27.
McKeganey, N. (1984a), 'Rudolf Steiner's anthroposophy and curative education: the possibility of an adequate ethnography', *International*

Journal of Sociology and Social Policy, vol. 4, pp. 1–14.
McKeganey, N. (1984b), 'A comparison of therapeutic work in two therapeutic communities located within psychiatric hospitals', Institute of Medical Sociology Occasional Paper, no. 7, University of Aberdeen.
McKeganey, N. (1984c) 'No doubt she's really a little princess: a case study of trouble in a therapeutic community', *Sociological Review*, vol. 32, pp. 328–48.
McKeganey, N. (1986), 'Accomplishing ideals: the case of hospital-based therapeutic communities', *International Journal of Therapeutic Communities*, vol. 7, pp. 85–100.
McKeganey, N. and Bloor, M. (1987), 'Teamwork, information control and therapeutic effectiveness', *Sociology of Health and Illness*, vol. 9, pp. 155–78.
McKeganey, N. and Cunningham-Burley, S. (eds) (1987), *Enter the Sociologist: Reflections on the Practice of Sociology*, Avebury, Gower.
McMichael, P. (1972), 'Loaningdale approved school: a study of the impact of an experimental regime on its boys', Godfrey Thomson Unit for Academic Assessment, University of Edinburgh.
Main, T. F. (1946), 'The hospital as a therapeutic institution', *Bulletin of the Menninger Clinic*, vol. 10, pp. 66–87.
Manning, N. (1976a), 'Innovation in social policy – the case of the therapeutic community', *Journal of Social Policy*, vol. 5, pp. 265–79.
Manning, N. (1976b), 'Values and practice in the therapeutic community', *Human Relations*, vol. 29, pp. 125–38.
Manning, N. and Blake, R. (1979), 'Implementing ideals' in R. D. Hinshelwood and N. Manning (eds), *Therapeutic Communities: Reflections and Progress*, London, Routledge & Kegan Paul.
Martin, D. (1972), 'The therapeutic community treatment of neurosis', in E. Schoenberg (ed.), *A Hospital Looks at Itself: Essays from Claybury*, London, Classics.
Marx, K. (1963), *Early Writings*, (ed. and trans. T. Bottomore), London, Watts.
Mead, G. H. (1934), *Mind, Self and Society*, Chicago, University of Chicago Press.
Mehan, B. and Wood, H. (1975), *The Reality of Ethnomethodology*, New York, Wiley.
Morrice, J. K. (1965), 'Permissiveness', *British Journal of Medical Psychology*, vol. 38, pp. 247–56.
Morrice, J. K. (1968), 'The community as therapist', *Journal of the Fort Logan Mental Health Care Centre*, vol. 4, pp. 125–47.
Morrice, J. K. (1972), 'Myth and the democratic process', *British Journal of Medical Psychology*, vol. 45, pp. 237–46.
Morrice, J. K. (1973), 'A day hospital's function in a mental health service', *British Journal of Psychiatry*, vol. 122, pp. 307–14.
Morrice, J. K. (1979), 'Basic concepts, a critical review', in R. Hinshelwood and N. Manning (eds), *Therapeutic Communities: Reflections and Progress*, London, Routledge & Kegan Paul.
Myers, K. (1979), 'The mental hospital therapeutic community in recent years' in R. Hinshelwood and N. Manning (eds), *Therapeutic*

Communities: Reflections and Progress, London, Routledge & Kegan Paul.

Myers, K. and Clark, D. (1972), 'Results in a therapeutic community', *British Journal of Psychiatry*, vol. 120, pp. 51–8.

Navarro, V. (1976), 'The industrialisation of fetishism or the fetishism of industrialisation, a critique of Ivan Illich', *International Journal of Health Services*, vol. 5, pp. 351–71.

Oakley, A. (1981), 'Interviewing women: a contradiction in terms' in H. Roberts (ed.), *Doing Feminist Research*, London, Routledge & Kegan Paul.

Ofshe, R., Berg, N., Caughlin, R., Dolinajec, G., Gerson, K. and Johnson, A. (1974), 'Social structure and social control in Synanon', *Journal of Voluntary Action Research*, vol. 3, pp. 67–76.

Orford, J., Hawker, A. and Nicholls, P. (1974), 'An investigation of an alcoholism rehabilitation halfway house: I, Types of client and modes of discharge, *British Journal of the Addictions*, vol. 69, pp. 213–24.

Parsons, T. (1964), *The Structure of Social Action*, New York, Free Press.

Pollner, M. (1975), 'The very coinage of your brain: the anatomy of reality disjunctures', *Philosophy of the Social Sciences*, vol. 5, pp. 411–30.

Pollner, M. and Emerson, R. (1983), 'The dynamics of inclusion and distance in fieldwork relations', in R. Emerson (ed.), *Contemporary Field Research, a Collection of Readings*, Boston, Little Brown.

Polsky, H. (1962), *Cottage Six: The Social System of Delinquent Boys in Treatment*, New York, Russell Sage.

Psathas, G. (1968), 'Ethnomethods and phenomenology', *Social Research*, vol. 35, pp. 500–20.

Rapoport, R. (1960), *Community as Doctor*, London, Tavistock.

Raskin, D. (1971), 'Problems in the therapeutic community', *American Journal of Psychiatry*, vol. 128, pp. 492–4.

Rawlings, B. (1980), 'Everyday therapy: a study of routine practices in a therapeutic community', unpublished PhD thesis, University of Manchester.

Rawlings, B. (1981), 'Two practical concerns for therapists: the problems of real therapeutic communities and of success rates' in P. Atkinson and C. Heath (eds), *Medical Work, Realities and Routines*, London, Gower.

Reyes, A. (1983), 'Regression in a therapeutic community', unpublished MS.

Rigby, A. (1974), *Alternative Realities: A Study of Communes and their Members*, London, Routledge & Kegan Paul.

Rogers, C. (1951), 'A theory of personality and behaviour', in *Client Centred Therapy*, London, Constable.

Roosens, E. (1979), *Mental patients in town life: Geel – Europe's First Therapeutic Community*, Beverley Hills, Sage.

Rosenthal, M. (1980), 'Therapeutic community models: III, Phoenix House (USA)', in E. Jansen (ed.), *The Therapeutic Community*, London, Croom Helm.

Roth, J. (1963), *Timetables*, Chicago, Bobbs-Merrill.

Schutz, A. (1962a), *Collected Papers Volume I: The Problem of Social Reality*, (M. Natanson, ed.) The Hague, Nijhoff.

Schutz, A. (1962b), 'Commonsense and scientific interpretation of human action' in A. Schutz, *Collected Papers Volume I*, The Hague, Nijhoff.

Schutz, A. (1964a) *Collected Papers Volume II: Studies in Social Theory* (A. Brodersen ed.), The Hague, Nijhoff.

Schutz, A. (1964b), 'The homecomer' in A. Schutz, *Collected Papers Volume II*, The Hague, Nijhoff.

Schutz, A. (1964c), 'The social world and the theory of social action' in A. Schutz, *Collected Papers Volume II*, The Hague, Nijhoff.

Schutz, A. (1970), *Reflections on the Problem of Relevance*, (ed. R. Zaner), New Haven, Yale University Press.

Schutz, A. and Luckmann, T. (1974), *The Structure of the Life-World*, London, Heinemann.

Scull, A. (1977), *Decarceration: Community Treatment and the Deviant – a Radical View*, Englewood Cliffs, Free Press.

Scull, A. (1979), *Museums of Madness*, London, Allen Lane.

Sedgwick, P. (1982), *Psycho Politics*, London, Pluto Press.

Sharp, V. (1975), *Social Control in the Therapeutic Community*, Farnborough, Saxon House.

Smith, D. (1978), 'K. is mentally ill', *Sociology*, vol. 12, pp. 23–53.

Srole, L. (1977), 'Geel, Belgium – the natural therapeutic community', in G. Serban and B. Astrachan (eds), *New Trends of Psychiatry in the Community*, Cambridge, Ballinger.

Steiner, R. (1928), *The Story of my Life*, New York, Anthroposophical Publishing.

Steiner, R. (1958), *The Three-fold Social Order*, New York, Anthroposophical Publishing.

Steiner, R. (1972), *Lectures on Curative Education*, London, Rudolf Steiner Press.

Strauss, A., Fagerhaugh, S., Suczek, B. and Wiener, C. (1985), *Social Organisation of Medical Work*, London, University of Chicago Press.

Strong, P. (1979), *The Ceremonial Order of the Clinic*, London, Routledge & Kegan Paul.

Sugarman, B. (1974), *Daytop Village, a Therapeutic Community*, New York, Holt, Rinehart and Winston.

Sugarman, B. (1975), 'Reluctant converts: social control, socialisation and adaptation in therapeutic communities', in R. Wallis (ed.), *Sectarianism*, London, Peter Owen.

Tizard, J., Sinclair, I. and Clarke, R. (1975), Introduction in Tizard et al. (eds), *Varieties of Residential Experience*, London, Routledge & Kegan Paul.

Volkman, R. and Cressey, D. R. (1963), 'Differential association and the rehabilitation of drug addicts', *American Journal of Sociology*, vol. 64, pp. 129–42.

Walter, J. A. (1978), *Sent Away: A Study of Young Offenders in Care*, Farnborough, Saxon House.

Warnock, E. (1978), *Report on Special Educational Needs*, Department of Education and Science, London, HMSO.

Wartofsky, M. (1974), 'Organs, organisms and disease: human ontology and medical practice', in H. Engelhert and S. Spicker (eds), *Evaluation*

and Explanation in the Biomedical Sciences, Boston, D. Reidel.
Weihs, A. (1965), 'The Camphill movement and the Camphill School', *Cresset*, vol. 11 no. 3, pp. 155–67.
Weihs, T. (1971), *Children in Need of Special Care*, London, Souvenir Press.
Weihs, T. (1975), 'The handicapped child – curative education', in J. Davy (ed.), *Work Arising*, London, Rudolf Steiner Press.
Wells, M. (1980), 'Therapeutic Community Models: I, Spring Lake Ranch (U.S.A.)', in E. Jansen (ed.), *The Therapeutic Community*, London, Croom Helm.
Whiteley, J. S. and Gordon, J. (1979), *Group Approaches in Psychiatry*, London, Routledge & Kegan Paul.
Whyte, W. F. (1955), *Street Corner Society* (second edition), Chicago, University of Chicago Press.
Wiener, C., Strauss, A. Fagerhaugh, S. and Suczek, B. (1979), 'Trajectories, biographies, and the evolving medical scene, labour and delivery and the intensive care nursery', *Sociology of Health and Illness*, vol. 1, pp. 261–83.
Wills, W. D. (1941), *The Hawkspur Experiment*, London, Allen & Unwin.
Wills, W. D. (1964), *Homer Lane – a Biography*, London, Allen & Unwin.
Wills, W. D. (1971), *Spare the Child*, Harmondsworth, Penguin.
Wilson, S. and Mandelbrote, B. (1978), 'Factors related to criminal activity after treatment in a therapeutic community for drug dependence', *British Journal of Criminology*, vol. 132, pp. 84–97.
Wing, J. (1957), 'Family care systems in Norway and Holland', *Lancet*, ii, pp. 884–6.
Wing, J. (1978), *Reasoning about Madness*, London, Oxford University Press.
Wootton, A. (1977), 'Sharing: some notes on the organisation of talk in a therapeutic community', *Sociology*, vol. 11, pp. 333–50.
World Health Organisation (1953), *Third Report of Expert Committee on Mental Health*, Geneva WHO.
Yabbusky, L. (1965), The Tunnel Back, New York, Macmillan.
Zeitlyn, B. (1967), 'The therapeutic community – fact or fantasy', *British Journal of Psychiatry*, vol. 113, pp. 1083–6.

Name Index

Subject Index

69 5

69 5